REVISED STANDARDS AND GUIDELINES OF SERVICE

for the Library of Congress Network of Libraries for the Blind and Physically Handicapped

2011

ASSOCIATION OF SPECIALIZED AND COOPERATIVE LIBRARY AGENCIES

AMERICAN LIBRARY ASSOCIATION

CHICAGO, 2011

© 2012

Published by the Association of Specialized and Cooperative Library Agencies

American Library Association
50 East Huron Street
Chicago, Illinois 60611

ISBNs: 978-0-8389-8595-3 (paper); 978-0-8389-9381-1 (PDF).

The paper used in this publication meets the minimum requirements of American National Standard for Information Sciences—Permanence of Paper for Printed Library Materials. ANSI 239.48-1984. ∞

© 2012 by the American Library Association. Any claim of copyright is subject to applicable limitations and exceptions, such as rights of fair use and library copying pursuant to Sections 107 and 108 of the U.S. Copyright Act. No copyright is claimed for content in the public domain, such as works of the U.S. government.

Printed in the United States of America.

Working Team

Jill Lewis, Maryland State Library for the Blind and Physically Handicapped

Mike Marlin, California Braille and Talking Book Library

Tom Peters (Project Director), TAP Information Services

Stephen Prine (ex officio), Library of Congress National Library Service for the Blind and Physically Handicapped

Advisory Team

Stephen Prine, Library of Congress National Library Service for the Blind and Physically Handicapped

Will Reed, Ohio Library for the Blind & Physically Disabled

Stella Cone, Georgia Libraries for Accessible Statewide Services

Margaret Conroy, representing the Chief Officers of State Library Agencies (COSLA)

Kim Charlson, representing the American Council of the Blind

Claudia Perry, representing the Blinded Veterans Association

David Hyde, representing the National Federation of the Blind

Mike Marlin (ex officio), California Braille and Talking Book Library

Jill Lewis (ex officio), Maryland State Library for the Blind and Physically Handicapped

Tom Peters (ex officio), TAP Information Services

Contents

Foreword 1

Acknowledgments 9

Introduction 10

Standards

    1.   Provision of Services 14

    2.   Resource Development and Management 21

    3.   Public Education and Outreach 25

    4.   Consulting Services 26

    5.   Volunteers and Internship Programs 28

    6.   Administration and Organization 29

    7.   Budget and Funding 30

    8.   Planning and Evaluation 31

    9.   Policies and Procedures 32

    10.   Reports 34

    11.   Personnel 34

    12.   Research and Development 36

    13.   BARD (Braille and Audio Reading Download) 37

Guidelines

    1. Personnel 39

    2. Space 42

Glossary 44

Appendices

A. Statement of Principles and Considerations 55

B. LC/NLS Service Eligibility Criteria 60

C. Lending Agency Service Agreement for Sound Reproducers and Other Reading Equipment 62

D. Pratt-Smoot Act and Major Amendments 71

E. ALA Library Bill of Rights and Policy on Confidentiality of Library Records 74

F. ALA Policy on Services for People with Disabilities 76

Index 80

Foreword

History

The Library of Congress National Library Service for the Blind and Physically Handicapped (LC/NLS) cooperative network includes fifty-six regional libraries, forty-seven subregional libraries, four separate machine-lending agencies, two multistate centers, and LC/NLS itself. The goal of this network is to serve eligible readers and is the result of more than one hundred years of development and experience.

Before the turn of the twentieth century, library service for blind people was initiated by a number of public libraries throughout the United States. The Boston Public library established a department for the blind in 1868 after receiving eight embossed volumes. Between 1882 and 1903 public libraries in Philadelphia, Chicago, New York City, and Detroit established circulating collections of embossed books for the blind. New York was the first state to create a department for blind in a state library.

During the same period the concept of a national library for the blind was developed in 1897 by John Russell Young, Librarian of Congress, when he established a reading room with about five hundred books and music items in raised type. In 1913 Congress provided that one copy of each book in raised type made for educational purposes under government subsidy by the American Printing House for the Blind in Louisville, Kentucky, was to be deposited in the Library of Congress. Other materials were acquired by gift and purchase.

These early steps led to the Library of Congress National Library Service for the Blind and Physically Handicapped (LC/NLS), which came into existence with the enactment of the Pratt-Smoot Act on March 3, 1931. The Pratt-Smoot Act mandated that the Librarian of Congress provide books for the use of adult blind residents of the United States, including the states, territories, insular possessions, and the District of Columbia. It also authorized the Librarian of Congress to make arrangements with other appropriate libraries to serve as local or regional centers for circulating these books. Nineteen libraries were selected to participate, forming one of the first "national networks" of libraries in t he United States.

A 1933 amendment to the act expanded the service to include books on records, which precipitated establishment of an additional seven regional libraries. The network remained at twenty-six regional libraries until 1950 when a regional library was established in Florida. Expansion continued through the 1960s and 1970s, the late 1960s seeing the first subregional libraries, a concept that spread across the country in the 1970s and first half of the 1980s. Regional library expansion continued until 1976 with the establishment of regional libraries in Alaska and Vermont. The network consisted of fifty-six regional libraries until the North Dakota State Library established a regional library in 1995. In 2009, the southern Ohio regional library closed and the service was picked up by the regional library serving northern Ohio. Subregional library expansion continued until the mid 1980s when expansion peaked and then began to decline.

In the years since 1931, there have been a number of significant additions and changes in the services offered. In 1952, the word "adult" was deleted to allow services to blind children. In 1962, music services were added and in 1966, the act was amended again to extend library service to physically handicapped individuals.

Also beginning in the mid 1960s the Library Services and Construction Act (LSCA) authorized libraries to use federal funds distributed through state libraries to serve blind and physically handicapped persons; this change was a catalyst for the network library migration to automated circulation systems, the development of additional services, and in some states the establishment of subregional libraries.

Development of Standards

This edition of the Standards is the most recent in a series of standards dealing with library service for the network of cooperating libraries serving blind and physically handicapped individuals. The development of standards for this service began over fifty years ago in 1957 when the American Foundation for the Blind commissioned and published Francis R. St. John's *Survey of Library Services for the Blind 1956* (1). It summarized the state of the art as it existed in 1956, contained recommendations for the future development of library service for the blind, and established the need for a set of basic standards.

St. John's recommendation for the development of basic standards for library service for the blind led in 1961 to the development of *Standards for Regional Libraries for the Blind* (2). This cooperative venture of the Library of Congress Division for the Blind and the American Library Association (ALA) Round Table on Library Services to the Blind resulted in a five-page mimeographed publication with a modest statement of goals.

In 1965-66 a Committee on Standards for Library Services of the Commission on Standards and Accreditation of Services for the Blind, later the National Accreditation Council, developed standards. Ralph R. Shaw served as chair, Lowell A. Martin as vice-chair. These standards were for all types of libraries at the federal, state, and community levels, as well as for school libraries and libraries for agencies serving blind and visually handicapped persons. They were adopted by the American Library Association in 1967 (3).

In 1977, the successor to the ALA Round Table for the Blind, the Library Services to the Blind and Physically Handicapped (LSBPH) Section of the Health and Rehabilitative Library Services Division (HRLSD) of ALA, appointed a committee to draft new standards for library service for blind and physically handicapped individuals. The members of HRLSD and the committee agreed that standards were needed not only for the national network of libraries serving the blind and physically handicapped, but also for the services provided for this group by all types of libraries. However, they decided to focus on the LC/NLS network in the initial phase of standards development and to encourage the development in the future of guidelines or standards for the related services in state library agencies, public libraries, elementary and secondary school libraries, academic libraries, special libraries, and libraries in institutions such as hospitals, nursing homes, and correctional facilities. LC/NLS funded the development of the first edition of the standards through a contract with HRLSD, and the project began in September 1977.

The first *Standards* were approved by the Board of Directors of the Association of Specialized and Cooperative Library Agencies (ASCLA), formally HRLSD and ASLA, a division of the American Library Association, on January 7, 1979. At the time, the ASCLA Standards for Library Service to the Blind and Physically Handicapped Subcommittee recommended that the implementation of the standards be monitored with the goal of formulating new standards within five years.

In 1980, LC/NLS contracted with Battelle Columbus Laboratories (Battelle) to conduct several activities associated with the standards. Among them was a study comparing the regional libraries in the network and LC/NLS against the 1979 standards. This study, called the standards survey, resulted in individual detailed reports for each regional library, LC/NLS and its multistate centers, as well as an executive summary describing national findings in general. Battelle also was charged with recommending an ongoing process for monitoring network libraries' success in meeting the existing standards. The standards survey was completed in December 1982.

By 1982, conditions were favorable for the revision of the 1979 Standards as recommend by the ASCLA Standards for Library Service for the Blind and Physically Handicapped Subcommittee. The Battelle standards survey and the activity of the ASCLA Standards Subcommittee (charged with monitoring the implementation of the 1979 standards) resulted in information about the need for revision of the Standards as well as the extent and nature of the revision process. In fact, no other known set of national library standards had been examined so thoroughly and tested so quickly in the field. The findings of the various studies and the opinion of network practitioners emphasized the need to revise the *Standards*.

Aware of the need for a new standards document, ASCLA submitted to LC/NLS in 1982 a proposal for a contract to revise the *Standards for the Library of Congress Network of Libraries for the Blind and Physically Handicapped*. LC/NLS awarded the contract to ASCLA in November 1982.

The 1984 standards provided network libraries, state library agencies, administering and funding agencies with a useful tool for assessing the current status of library services for blind and physically handicapped persons. In addition, they provided standards of service to be achieved and guidelines for achieving specific standards. The importance of planning and evaluation as a basis of providing and assessing library services is emphasized.

These standards were adopted by the Board of Directors of the Association of Specialized and Cooperative Library Agencies (ASCLA), a division of ALA, in January 1984.

ASCLA has a policy of reviewing standards every five years. However, funding and community interest did not come together until 1991, when informal discussion about revision were moved forward with LC/NLS indicating to the ASCLA Standards Review Committee its willingness to again support a process to revise the standards. The ASCLA Standards Review Committee, after determining that the 1984 standards would benefit from revision, submitted a proposal for financial support to LC/NLS. These standards were adopted by the ASCLA Board of Directors in February 1995.

The 1995 document reflected the fundamental changes to the environment in which these services are provided, resulting primarily from the impact and effects of technological advances and from the passage of the Americans with Disabilities Act (ADA). The document recognized that local conditions, always varied, could now have even more significant variations from agency to agency. In addition, the document reflected the awareness that conditions at each level of service are more volatile, that the final effects of major influences such as ADA and technology are not yet known, and that changes will continue to occur with increasing rapidity.

After these standards were used for eight years, the ASCLA Standards Review Committee recommended that the standards be revised again. In discussions with ASCLA, LC/NLS agreed to underwrite the cost of bringing appropriate parties together to expedite the process. The contract was signed in 2003 and with the selection of a project director by ASCLA the project began in the summer of 2003. Public discussion sessions were held at ALA annual conferences in Toronto and Orlando and the midwinter conference in San Diego. The project director attended and spoke at the NLS national conference in Rapid City, South Dakota in May 2004. Two drafts were circulated for comments and the final draft was taken to the ALA midwinter meeting in Boston and was approved by the ASCLA Board of Directors.

LC/NLS and the network agreed that with the transition from an analog to a digital format, the standards should once again be updated. ASCLA submitted a proposal and a contract was signed in December 2009. This new iteration of the standards, published in the fall of 2011, has three distinct changes from previous the standards. First, is the inclusion of standards relating to the use of interns. Second, the addition of a new section of standards relating to the Braille and Audio Reading Download (BARD). BARD was developed and is maintained by the National Library Service for the Blind and Physically Handicapped (LC/NLS) for use by eligible readers who have access to the Internet and to the network of cooperating libraries. This Web site holds a collection of all audio titles physically produced in digital format since 2008, and all audio titles for which LC/NLS has a digital master or will convert to digital format from an analog format. The site also contains downloadable copies of audio magazines being produced on analog cassette. All audio, future braille titles, and existing web-braille titles will be mounted on BARD once they have passed quality assurance. The site enables both readers and network libraries to download titles from the LC/NLS national collection for personal reading pleasure by the reader or as a master for duplication of additional copies if so needed by a network library. Third, a revision, the first since the 1979 standards, of the guidelines relating to staffing levels at regional and subregional libraries.

This revision identifies the goals which the community agrees should be met in provision of this library service and establishes the foundation upon which the next iteration of these standards will be built.

Structure of the National Network

The structure of the national network of libraries providing library service for blind and physically handicapped persons contributes to the development of local enhancements to the basic program. As with earlier versions, an understanding of that structure helps to clarify the purpose and scope of these standards. Currently, the major components of the network are the Library of Congress, National Library Service for the Blind and Physically Handicapped and its Multistate Centers (MSC), regional and subregional libraries, separate machine-lending agencies, and their respective administering and funding agencies.

The standards cover those for which LC/NLS, regional and subregional libraries are responsible. Within the network, network libraries and their administrative and funding agencies have a variety of contractual arrangements for the provision of goods and services. Where those services, products, or processes are those named in these standards, the contracting agencies are expected to comply with the standards.

Within the standards, when the phrase, "network libraries" is used, it is applicable to LC/NLS, regional libraries and subregional libraries. Where a standard is specific to one of these, that is so stated.

No network library is a wholly independent agency. Each has an administrating agency of which the network library is a unit. In the case of LC/NLS, that administrating agency is the Library of Congress. The administrating agency of a regional library may be a state library or agency, a public library, a commission for the blind, a state department of education, or a private service agency. At present, all but two subregional libraries are a unit of a public library or library system. The other two are administered by schools for the blind.

The agency that funds the regional or subregional library may be the administering agency. In other cases, the funding agency and the administering agency are different agencies. While the singularity or combination of administering and funding agencies vary from state to state, in all cases the network library follows the administrative policies and procedures of its administering agency. In all cases, local law, ordinances, contract or labor agreement take precedent over the standards.

The state library agency may or may not have a direct or formal relationship to the administering or funding agencies or to the regional or subregional libraries in its service area. Because it is responsible for overall library service and development in the state, however, the state library agency always has an indirect or advisory relationship with agencies administering, funding, or providing library service to blind and physically handicapped persons even where no formal, direct relationship exits.

Various local elements contribute to the development of enhancements to the basic service at the regional and subregional levels. The nature of the administrative or funding agency, the structure of services in the state, and the level or variety of local resources are among the controlling factors. The variety of locally developed services is infinite and precludes the standards addressing any specificity. More appropriately, the standards emphasize the importance of developing these enhancements to the basic service.

Services in addition to providing LC/NLS-generated recorded

materials, braille, and music materials are closely associated with the network, in providing for a population that includes those who are eligible for basic network services. Among these are radio reading services, dial-in newspapers, large-print materials, descriptive videos, and commercial sound or spoken-word recordings. The provision or administration of these associated services is not universally the responsibility of regional or subregional libraries. In some cases, these services are provided through separate and independent agencies and in other cases, they are a traditional service provided to the general community by the local public library. Because these services are not always provided through network libraries, but sometimes are part of the traditional services of non-network agencies, they also are not included in these standards.

---

1. Francis R. St. John, *Survey of Library Service for the Blind*, 1956 (New York: American Foundation for the Blind, 1957)

2. American Library Association, Round Table on Library Service to the Blind, *Standards for Regional Libraries for the Blind*, mimeographed (Washington, D.C.: Division for the Blind, Library of Congress, 1961) 5pp.

3. American Library Association, Library Administration Division, *Standards for Library Services for the Blind and Visually Handicapped* (Chicago: ALA, 1967)

Acknowledgments

Revising these standards and guidelines would have been very difficult without the talents and efforts of many individuals and groups, past and present. Communication methods included in-person and online meetings and forums, conference calls, and numerous email messages.

The members of the advisory team gave freely of their time, experiences, and insights into each phase of the process of revising these standards and guidelines. They sought and duly considered feedback from a wide variety of individuals and groups. They spent many long hours in the Judith Krug Room at ALA headquarters in Chicago discussing big ideas, complex issues, pointed criticisms, and minute details. Their commitment to making these standards and guidelines viable for at least the next ten years supports the network goal of providing consistently excellent services to all eligible users.

Susan Hornung and her staff at ASCLA were very adept and thoughtful in supporting this project. They handled all the fiscal matters, local arrangements, and much more. Their contributions and commitment to this process enabled the members of the Working Team and Advisory Team to concentrate on the actual revisions work with minimal distractions.

Everyone involved in the current project also thanks everyone who contributed to previous iterations of these standards and guidelines, particularly Courtney Deines-Jones, the project director of the revisions process that resulted in the 2005 Standards and Guidelines, as well as all members of the Working Team and Advisory Committee. Without their hard work and thoughtful deliberations, our task would have been much more arduous.

Introduction by Tom Peters, Project Director

The Revised Standards and Guidelines of Service for the Library of Congress Network of Libraries for the Blind and Physically Handicapped, 2011, continues the tradition of fruitful collaboration between ASCLA and LC/NLS to develop, hone, and promulgate these standards and guidelines. The current project, building on the 2005 revised standards, began with an RFP process to select a project director and the appointment of members to the working team and the advisory team to help guide the process and to provide ongoing input into the standards and guidelines from diverse stakeholder organizations and individuals.

Members of the Working Team and the Advisory Team met in person in Chicago in April 2010 to develop an overall process and timeline for this project, and to draft a statement of principles and considerations. A public draft of the statement of principles and considerations was released on May 7, 2010. Based on comments made to the first draft statement of principles and considerations, as well as on further discussion by the project teams, a revised statement of principles and considerations was released on June 28, 2010.

A public forum was held in June 2010 in conjunction with the ALA Annual Conference held in Washington, DC. The Working Team and Advisory Team received many valuable comments and suggestions during that forum and via other communication with stakeholders, and continued working on preliminary revisions to the standards and guidelines. The first public drafts of the proposed revised standards and guidelines were released in December 2010.

A second public forum was held in January 2011 both in-person and online in conjunction with the ALA Midwinter Meeting in San Diego. Again we received an excellent, thoughtful batch of public comments, each of which were duly considered by the project teams. On April 4, 2011 a second public draft of the proposed revised standards and guidelines was released. Another round of online and in-person forums ensued in April and May, several in conjunction with the regional conferences. On May 23-24 the members of the working and advisory teams met again at ALA Headquarters in Chicago to review and discuss all of the comments and suggestions that were made in response to the second public draft.

An online archive of this process, including the progression of the various versions of the documents, as well as recordings of the online forums, can be found at http://www.tapinformation.com/ASCLANLS.htm.

Any standards initiative, like many endeavors, involves both a process and a product. Actually, there are two clusters of processes: Those that occur before the publication and dissemination of the standards, and those that occur after publication and dissemination, as interested organizations and individuals interpret and apply the standards and guidelines.

The Purpose of This Document

These standards and guidelines are intended to help LC/NLS network libraries maintain the best service levels for eligible individuals and organizations. The scope is similar to that represented in the 2005, 1995, and earlier versions of these standards and guidelines. The goal is to provide appropriate service standards for the development and deployment of LC/NLS network library services and activities, including direct patron services, collection development and management, outreach efforts, the production of local materials, and more. These standards and guidelines have been crafted to reflect a level of excellence that we, the members of the Working Team and the Advisory Team, believe the LC/NLS user population deserves, and to which all network libraries can aspire.

These standards and guidelines address standards of service. To the greatest extent possible we have focused on the goals and outcomes of an action, rather than on the specific means to achieve an articulated outcome. By doing this, we hope that the document will remain pertinent for at least ten years.

The guidelines, especially regarding staffing levels, have been updated, based in part on the results of a staffing survey administered to regional and subregional libraries during the fall of 2010.

For Whom This Document Is Intended

Staff members, volunteers, members of advisory groups, parent organizations, stakeholder groups, and users of LC/NLS network library services should use this set of standards and guidelines to review and analyze services as part of assessment and strategic planning initiatives. Equal consideration should be given to areas where service could be improved and to areas where the standards are being met or exceeded.

Users of the service can use this document as a guide to better understand the goals, breadth, and depth of the service goals of the LC/NLS network. Please note that administrative structures, funding sources, operating plans and procedures, and other support provided to network libraries vary from state to state. These variations can affect a library's ability to meet service standards. Users of the LC/NLS service can be powerful advocates for improved services – by volunteering to serve on advisory groups, by lobbying for increased funding, or by becoming involved in friends groups and similar initiatives.

Representatives of stakeholder organizations, agencies, and groups are encouraged to use this document as an educational and awareness tool, and as a way to assess how the library services available to their constituents compare against the recommended standards and guidelines. Again, stakeholder organizations, agencies, and groups should collaborate with network libraries to promote the use of LC/NLS services among eligible individuals, and to improve service delivery.

Representatives of administrative and funding agencies are encouraged to use this document as a planning tool to identify both best practices areas and those areas that might benefit from procedural improvements and better resource allocations and commitments. The standards also can be used as one measure of how well library services in a particular state, territory, district, or region compare against these recommended national standards.

Members of agencies and organizations serving potential users of LC/NLS services, such as public libraries, retirement communities, nursing homes, assisted living services, and schools serving students who have print disabilities, should use this document as an awareness and educational tool. LC/NLS network services can significantly improve and enhance the quality of life for participating eligible individuals.

Ways to Use This Document

We recommend that all individuals and groups involved in providing, funding, or administering network library services use this document in the following ways:

1. First, review all of the sections (or, for those involved in only selected service areas, the relevant sections) of the standards to become familiar with the structure and substance of the standards of recommended service. To make the standards as concise as possible, nearly all facets are listed only once at the point in the structure of the standards that makes the most sense.

2. Next, examine the guidelines, because they provide a basic reference and benchmark to the space, staffing, and shelving resources needed to provide excellent service.

3. Identify service areas in which you believe your library is meeting or exceeding the standards, as well as those areas where

improvement may be a goal. Also identify any standards that are not applicable to your particular institution.

4. Briefly annotate the standards, using either the margins of the print publication or the digital version, paying special attention to areas where the library is meeting or exceeding expectations, where improvement is indicated, and where standards are not deemed applicable.

5. Focusing on the service goals advanced by these standards, prioritize areas for improvement with input from all stakeholder groups and assistance as needed from regional or national LC/NLS consultants.

6. Use this prioritized list as one of the primary inputs for strategic planning, for developing action plans for process and service improvements, and for requesting additional funding from the principal funding organization, foundations, grant-funding agencies, individual donors, and other sources of funding.

7. Use your analysis of the standards met or exceeded to develop and promote success stories, and to articulate best practices that can be shared with other member organizations of the LC/NLS network.

Additional Comments

The Working Team and the Advisory Team received many comments, questions, concerns, and recommendations about this project to revise these standards and guidelines. I am happy to report that the project teams duly considered every communication received. After due consideration, the Working Team and Advisory Team wove some of the substance of these communications into the standards and guidelines. For other communications, after some discussion and debate, the two teams decided not to incorporate the substance of a particular communication into the revised standards and guidelines. These exclusions do not necessarily mean that the two project teams disagreed with the comments or suggestions. Usually the decision to exclude something rested on the groups' sense of the scope of this set of standards and guidelines. Sometimes the two teams felt that the substance of a communication dealt primarily with how a standard or guideline should be implemented locally, which the two teams feel is a local decision and responsibility, made on the basis of local conditions and trends. Other suggestions (for example, the recommendation that NLS change its official name) were considered by the two teams to be beyond the pale of this particular revision process, but the two teams recommend that appropriate groups duly consider these larger suggestions and recommendations.

Standards

1. Provision of Services

    1.1   Network libraries and machine lending agencies (MLA) shall register patrons in compliance with PL 89-522 (Pratt-Smoot Act as amended and extended) (see Appendix D).

        a. In the lending of content, metadata, hardware, and software, preference shall be given at all times to the needs of blind and other eligible print-disabled persons who have been honorably discharged from the armed forces of the United States.

        b. Network libraries and machine lending agencies shall maintain information about patrons to meet LC/NLS requirements and to provide service, resulting in quantifiable information, while maintaining patron confidentiality.

        c. Network libraries and machine lending agencies shall, within 5 (five) business days of receiving an application for service, verify that the application is complete, initiate contact for additional information, or return the application for proper certification.

        d. Once a completed application is verified, network libraries and machine lending agencies shall initiate service within 2 (two) business days.

        e. Network libraries and machine lending agencies that have in their service areas schools serving eligible children shall contact these schools to make every effort to ensure that all eligible children in the schools are registered for LC/NLS services.

        f. Network libraries and machine lending agencies shall ensure the confidentiality of patron records, following applicable laws as well as the guidelines presented in the ALA Policy on Confidentiality of Library Records (see

Appendix E).

1.2 Machine lending agencies and sublending agencies (SLA) shall comply with the MLA agreements and the sublending agency agreement.

    a. LC/NLS shall provide each MLA and SLA with a procedures manual.

    b. Network libraries, MLAs, and SLAs shall provide playback equipment and accessories within 2 (two) business days of a patron request.

    c. As developed and made available, network libraries shall provide playback equipment and accessories using an equitable distribution policy, taking into consideration that federal law gives preference to veterans and NLS policy gives secondary preference to centenarians (10 Squared members).

1.3 Network libraries and machine lending agencies shall maintain all circulation and machine lending data electronically, including BARD circulation.

1.4 Network libraries may develop different loan periods for different formats.

    a. Network libraries shall levy no fine on overdue, damaged, or lost materials which are part of the LC/NLS national collection.

    b. Network libraries shall develop and communicate to their patrons appropriate loan policies for materials in the local collection, such as large print materials and descriptive videos.

1.5 Network libraries and machine lending agencies shall ensure convenient access to materials and services.

    a. Network libraries and machine lending agencies shall provide materials and information about these services in appropriate accessible formats.

b. Network libraries and machine lending agencies shall provide service during normal business hours.

c. Network libraries shall ensure that they meet reasonable preferences and service requests.

d. Network libraries shall provide reader advisors to assist patrons in identifying specific materials and formats in their areas of interest.

1.6 Network libraries and machine lending agencies shall provide services in languages other than English to the greatest extent possible and as appropriate to their communities. Network libraries shall maintain resources and collaborate with other institutions to serve patrons who speak or read languages other than English.

1.7 Network libraries and machine lending agencies shall facilitate and encourage various modes of independent access to materials and services. These models include, but are not limited to, accessible online catalogs, telephone, and other means. Network libraries shall develop and communicate processes and procedures for using these tools to all interested individuals and groups.

1.8 Network libraries and machine lending agencies shall process patron requests for materials and information within 5 (five) business days. Requests for books and magazines generated through *Talking Book Topics* or *Braille Book Review* and similar promotional activities shall be processed within 7 (seven) business days.

a. Network libraries and machine lending agencies shall have the capability to accept patron requests via toll-free voice including relay services for deaf callers, with toll-free telephone service that is answered by staff members during all business hours. During hours when the library is closed the toll-free number shall provide voice mail capability.

b. Network libraries and machine lending agencies shall offer patrons the option to make requests and receive service via online tools that are accessible.

   c. Network libraries and machine lending agencies shall have the capability to accept patron requests via fax and through the United States Postal Service (USPS).

   d. Network libraries and machine lending agencies shall have the capability to serve walk-in patrons.

1.9 Network libraries and machine lending agencies shall process all returned materials within 5 (five) business days.

   a. Network libraries shall ensure that circulating materials are inspected, in good condition, and fully prepared for the next patron.

1.10 Network libraries and machine lending agencies shall respond to patron requests for contact within 5 (five) business days.

1.11 Network libraries shall respond to patron requests for information, including reference requests.

   a. Network libraries shall fulfill ready reference requests from their patrons within 1 (one) business day.

   b. Network libraries shall fulfill in-depth reference requests from their patrons within 5 (five) business days.

   c. Network libraries shall collaborate, as appropriate, with libraries and other organizations to facilitate fulfillment of reference requests.

   d. Network libraries shall refer their patrons to public, university, and other libraries or resources when appropriate.

   e. Network libraries shall provide patrons with information about and referrals to other service agencies, when appropriate.

1.12 Network libraries shall provide newsletters at least quarterly and other direct communications as appropriate in accessible formats.

a. Network libraries shall have the capacity to deliver content in electronic formats.

b. Network libraries shall make electronic copies of newsletters and other direct communications available on a fully accessible Web site.

1.13 Network libraries shall maintain a fully accessible and usable public Web site, informed by the most recent guidelines issued by the Web Accessibility Initiative of the World Wide Web Consortium (W3C) (http://www.w3.org/WAI/).

a. Network library Web sites shall provide online public access catalogs (OPACs) and other appropriate bibliographic finding aids, including links to union catalogs.

b. Network libraries shall accept patron requests for materials and information via their Web sites or email.

c. Network libraries shall accept patron feedback via their Web sites or email.

d. Network libraries shall post electronic copies of all forms, patron policies and procedures; annual reports and other public documents; electronic copies of newsletters and other communications; hours of operation; links to LC/NLS; and other relevant information on their Web sites.

e. Network libraries shall frequently review all information and links on their Web sites to ensure information is current and correct.

f. Network libraries shall include supplemental information relevant to their patrons, such as links to consumer groups, other libraries, and service agencies, on their Web sites.

g. Network libraries providing Internet-based virtual reference services shall work to ensure that these services are fully accessible.

1.14 Network libraries shall maintain information about national, state, and local reading programs and book discussion groups and may facilitate patron participation in these community-based activities.

    a. Network libraries shall make bibliographies available to public and other libraries describing titles in the collection related to national, statewide, and regional reading program themes.

    b. Network libraries shall participate in national, regional, and/or local reading programs and book discussion groups.

    c. Network libraries may develop customized reading programs and book discussion groups as appropriate.

1.15 Network libraries shall promote storytelling and tactile resources for young (pre-reading) children through collaboration with public and other libraries, schools, and agencies promoting family literacy initiatives, early intervention programs, etc.

1.16 Network libraries shall provide appropriate special format materials and services developed by network libraries to serve all children and young adults.

1.17 Network libraries shall establish deposit collections and demonstration collections to extend services to eligible individuals who may reside in or are served by institutions.

1.18 Network libraries shall provide access to library materials through interlibrary loan or other resource sharing options within the United States.

1.19 LC/NLS shall coordinate alternative media book exchange and interlibrary loan with libraries and other agencies.

1.20 LC/NLS shall provide services to United States citizens residing abroad in compliance with these standards.

1.21 LC/NLS shall provide music service, such as braille and large print sheet music and instructional materials, directly to patrons in compliance with these standards.

1.22 LC/NLS shall provide direct service to patrons who need titles in obsolete, experimental, or little-used formats in compliance with these standards. Examples include TB, RD, and Grade 3 braille.

1.23 LC/NLS shall provide a fully accessible public Web site, informed by the most recent guidelines issued by the Web Accessibility Initiative of the World Wide Web Consortium (W3C) (http://www.w3.org/WAI/).

    a. LC/NLS shall provide access to the NLS international union catalog via the Web site.

    b. LC/NLS shall accept direct patron requests for music services.

    c. LC/NLS shall accept requests from U.S. citizens living abroad.

    d. LC/NLS shall accept and respond to patron feedback.

    e. LC/NLS shall post electronic copies of all forms, patron policies and procedures; annual reports and other public documents; electronic copies of newsletters and other communications; hours of operation; links to Network libraries; and other relevant information on a fully accessible Web site.

    f. LC/NLS shall periodically review all information and links on its Web site to ensure information is current and correct.

1.24 Network libraries shall acquire and maintain accurate patron name and address information on patrons being served and communicate: additions, deletions, and changes of address to the NLS Comprehensive Mailing List System (CMLS) vendor on a weekly basis.

2. Resource Development and Management

2.1 Network libraries shall acquire or produce reading materials to supplement the national collection as appropriate to their service communities.

   a. Network libraries that produce reading materials in specialized formats shall do so in accordance with appropriate copyright laws, in response to patron demand, and emphasizing titles of regional and local importance.

   b. Network libraries shall maintain original masters of all locally produced braille and/or recorded materials.

   c. Network libraries shall submit bibliographic information for locally produced titles to LC/NLS for inclusion in the international union catalog.

   d. Network libraries are encouraged to submit locally recorded materials to the MSCE Quality Assurance Program.

2.2 Network libraries that duplicate accessible format materials produced for the national collection shall do so according to LC/NLS quality control standards.

2.3 Network libraries shall maintain or provide access to collections of sufficient quantity and condition to meet patron demand in a timely and responsive manner.

   a. Network libraries shall alter or discontinue circulation of any format of material only with input from and in collaboration with LC/NLS, network library advisory groups, and patrons.

2.4 Network libraries shall develop and implement procedures to determine the number of copies of new titles to request from LC/NLS for the national collection.

   a. Regional libraries shall maintain, for audio titles available in a unique format and which are circulated, a minimum of one copy of each title they distribute that is provided by LC/NLS.

    b. Subregional libraries shall maintain in each format they circulate at least one copy of each title provided by LC/NLS in the preceding 24 (twenty-four) months.

    c. LC/NLS, in collaboration with network libraries, shall develop and implement appropriate retention policies for digital materials.

    d. Regional libraries shall ensure patrons have access to braille materials produced by LC/NLS.

2.5 Network libraries shall use the bibliographic standard adopted by LC/NLS when cataloging materials.

2.6 Network libraries shall, within their collection maintenance policies, systematically review and weed their collections, ensuring one copy is retained, in accordance with LC/NLS procedures.

2.7 Network libraries shall maintain information about national, state, and local organizations and programs concerned with services to eligible patrons.

2.8 Network libraries shall maintain or have access to professional materials and resources, in print or electronic formats, that support the development and provision of library services including a collection of standard reference works and of reader advisory reference materials.

2.9 LC/NLS shall develop directories and other appropriate tools to facilitate collaborations and resource sharing, and shall provide these publications electronically.

2.10 LC/NLS shall make available audio playback equipment and accessories.

    a. LC/NLS shall develop, maintain, and implement methods of quality control for LC/NLS-supplied audio playback equipment and accessories.

b. LC/NLS shall ensure, in cooperation with network libraries, equitable distribution of available playback equipment and accessories.

c. Network libraries and machine lending agencies shall maintain sufficient inventories to ensure provision of audio playback equipment and accessories within 5 (five) business days of a patron application or request.

2.11 LC/NLS shall develop and implement a systematic process of obtaining input from network librarians and patrons on the ongoing development of audio playback equipment and on equitable distribution methods for this equipment.

2.12 Network libraries shall maintain the capacity to download, duplicate, and circulate NLS audio books and magazines in digital format.

2.13 Network libraries shall maintain the capacity to duplicate and share locally produced digital braille files and/or digital audio files.

2.14 Network libraries shall participate in the NLS recall process for digital cartridges.

2.15 Network Libraries shall ensure equitable distribution of available equipment and accessories to patrons.

2.16 LC/NLS shall make available the national library collection.

a. LC/NLS shall continue to monitor and implement methods of quality control for materials added to the national collection.

b. LC/NLS shall, with network libraries, ensure equitable distribution of available materials.

c. LC/NLS shall provide a minimum of 2,000 audio titles and 475 braille titles annually.

2.17 LC/NLS shall continue to implement a systematic process of obtaining input from network libraries, advisory groups, and patrons on collection development and quantity of materials selected in addition to using standard collection development materials.

2.18 LC/NLS shall make available upon request in limited quantity other reading materials in accessible formats to supplement the national library collection, in addition to materials produced for distribution to the network. Examples of these materials include BRAs, BRFs, and RCFs.

2.19 LC/NLS shall continue to promulgate and monitor quality assurance standards for materials in accessible formats produced by network libraries.

    a. Network libraries shall meet LC/NLS quality assurance guidelines in producing accessible format materials to be added to the local collection.

    b. LC/NLS shall review locally produced materials submitted by network libraries to determine whether they meet LC/NLS quality assurance guidelines.

    c. LC/NLS shall facilitate the distribution of locally produced materials that meet LC/NLS quality assurance standards.

    d. Network libraries are encouraged to submit locally produced materials to the MSCE Quality Assurance Program.

2.20 LC/NLS shall provide network libraries with updated bibliographic information reflecting changes to the collection.

    a. LC/NLS shall continue to provide full bibliographic information in MARC 21 format for titles produced for the national collection, or the next generation of a delivery system.

    b. LC/NLS shall provide libraries and patrons with online access to a union catalog for all titles in the collection.

    c. LC/NLS shall, on a continuing basis, advise network

libraries of titles that LC/NLS has produced in quantity and titles that may be withdrawn from the collection.

    d.   Network libraries shall submit Intention and Completion Notices to LC/NLS for locally produced braille and/or digital audio titles for inclusion in the union catalog.

2.21 LC/NLS shall maintain a collection of titles in obsolete, experimental, or little-used formats.

2.22 LC/NLS shall maintain an archival collection of titles produced.

2.23 LC/NLS shall inform network libraries of basic and current professional literature pertaining to the physical conditions described in the LC/NLS eligibility requirements.

2.24 LC/NLS shall provide, in cooperation with network libraries, information pertaining to resources for, or of interest to, eligible patrons and shall make this resource information available in accessible formats.

3. Public Education and Outreach

3.1 Network libraries shall develop and implement a coordinated public awareness, education, and outreach plan for use in their service areas.

    a.   Network libraries shall collaborate with public and other libraries, schools, veterans' organizations, senior organizations, and other organizations and agencies as appropriate to promote their library services.

    b.   Network libraries shall develop and implement awareness programs and materials to reach students in library science, education, social service, and similar college and university programs as appropriate in their local service areas.

    c.   Network libraries shall conduct awareness activities and events as appropriate to promote a climate of public awareness favorable to the development, expansion, and improvement of library services. Examples include author and narrator events and open houses.

3.2 LC/NLS shall continually review network public awareness programs, and shall develop and implement national promotion, awareness, and education programs to effectively reach potential patrons. Examples include the anniversary of events such as the birth of Helen Keller or Louis Braille and the passage of the 1931 enabling legislation.

3.3 LC/NLS shall develop and disseminate a model for demographic analysis that can be adapted for use by network libraries.

   a. Network libraries and LC/NLS shall collaborate to conduct a demographic analysis based on the LC/NLS model.

4. Consulting Services

4.1 LC/NLS shall provide a minimum of 2 (two) full-time consultants to advise and assist network libraries.

   a. LC/NLS network consultants shall conduct biennial consulting visits to each regional library and machine lending agency.

   b. LC/NLS consultants shall prepare and submit a final written report of observations and recommendations and shall send a copy to the regional library or machine lending agency visited and its administering agency within 4 (four) months of the consultant visit.

   c. Visited regional libraries and machine lending agencies shall prepare a written response within 4 (four) months of receiving the consultant report and shall send a copy to their administering agency and the consultant.

   d. LC/NLS consultants shall call regional libraries in the off-year between visits to update the status of the recommendations from the last consultant report. Updates will be documented and sent to regional librarians, and the library's administering agency.

4.2 Regional libraries shall advise and assist subregional libraries as well as other libraries and agencies in the development and implementation of services in their geographic areas.

   a. Regional libraries shall conduct biennial consulting visits to each subregional library, according to LC/NLS procedures.

   b. Regional libraries shall prepare and submit a final written report of observations and recommendations and shall send a copy to the subregional library and its administering agency within 3 (three) months of the consultant visit.

   c. Visited subregional libraries shall prepare a written response within 3 (three) months of receiving the regional library report and shall send a copy to the LC/NLS regional consultant, administering agency, and the regional library.

4.3 Machine lending agencies shall advise and assist sublending agencies in the development and provision of services in their geographic areas.

   a. Machine lending agencies shall conduct biennial consulting visits to each sublending agency.

   b. Machine lending agencies shall prepare and submit a final written report of observations and recommendations and shall send a copy to the sublending agency, its administering agency, and LC/NLS within 3 (three) months of the machine lending agency visit.

   c. Visited sublending agencies shall prepare a written response within 3 (three) months of receiving the machine lending agency report and shall send a copy to their administering agency, the machine lending agency, and LC/NLS.

4.4 Subregional libraries shall advise and assist local libraries and related agencies in their geographic service areas.

4.5 Network libraries shall participate in networking through professional exchanges.

4.6 LC/NLS shall serve as a clearinghouse for information related to network services and operations.

5. Volunteers and Internship Programs

Volunteers

5.1 Network libraries and machine lending agencies shall, when permitted, use volunteers to assist in the performance of activities that supplement its basic program of services.

5.2 Network libraries and machine lending agencies shall not replace paid positions with volunteers.

5.3 Network libraries' and machine lending agencies' volunteer programs shall be managed in accordance with administering agency policy and practice.

5.4 Network libraries and machine lending agencies shall develop and implement an organizational structure that formally incorporates administration of the volunteer program.

5.5 Network libraries and machine lending agencies shall provide training, orientation programs, and materials for volunteers that include sensitivity to blindness and disabilities that qualify individuals to use this service, as well as the structure and philosophy of service.

5.6 Network libraries and machine lending agencies shall develop and implement programs that recognize volunteer activities at least annually.

5.7 Network libraries and machine-lending agencies shall work to identify new volunteer sources for equipment repair and other areas where additional support is needed.

Internship Programs

5.8 Network libraries and machine lending agencies shall use interns, when permitted, to assist in the performance of activities that supplement its basic program of service.

5.9 Network libraries and machine lending agencies shall not replace paid positions with interns.

5.10 Network libraries and machine lending agencies' intern program shall be managed in accordance with administering agency policy and practice, and those of the partner organizations, as appropriate.

5.11 Network libraries and machine lending agencies shall develop and implement an organizational structure that formally incorporates administration of the intern program.

5.12 Network libraries and machine lending agencies shall provide training, orientation programs and materials for interns that include sensitivity to blindness and disabilities that qualify individuals to use this service, as well as the structure and philosophy of the service.

5.13 Network libraries and machine lending agencies shall work to identify intern sources for areas where additional support is needed.

6. Administration and Organization

6.1. The state library agency or other administering agency shall be responsible for the development and coordination of this library service either directly through its administration and budget or indirectly through cooperation with the administering agency.

6.2. Each network library and machine lending agency shall comply with all laws and regulations pertaining to rights of and services to persons with disabilities.

6.3. The regional library shall be responsible for machine lending agency functions under their direction as described in the Lending Agency Service Agreement (Appendix C).

   a. The regional library or machine lending agency may

designate sublending agencies with LC/NLS concurrence.

  b. Each machine lending agency shall be responsible for ensuring that its sublending agencies comply with machine lending policy and procedure.

6.4 Network libraries shall administer, monitor, and evaluate deposit collections and demonstration collections' operation and service, while ensuring, at a minimum, an annual contact.

6.5 These Standards shall apply as appropriate to all network cooperating units, including contractors, institutional borrowers, and any others who perform services or functions covered in these Standards.

6.6 The network of cooperating libraries shall be composed of four regional conferences. Regional conferences should collaborate to sponsor joint meetings and events as appropriate.

6.7 Network libraries shall collect advice and input from a full spectrum of patrons and patron constituency groups through mechanisms including, but not limited to, advisory groups, focus groups, and patron forums that shall convene at least once a year. Network libraries shall make appropriate use of communications technologies to facilitate consumer participation in patron and patron constituency groups.

6.8 Network libraries shall, where applicable, support friends groups to promote library services.

6.9 Network library staff shall be encouraged to attend and present at consumer organizations and at other types of constituent gatherings and conferences to provide updates and information about Network programs and services.

7. Budget and Funding

7.1 Federal, state, and local units of government shall contribute funds, resources, and services to network libraries for the provision of library services to eligible patrons. Funds intended for seed funds, demonstration projects, and similar grants shall not be used to fund long-term ongoing operations.

7.2 Administering and funding agencies shall commit resources to enable network libraries and machine lending agencies to effectively operate, administer, and facilitate services as defined by these ASCLA Standards.

7.3 The head of each network library shall have primary responsibility for the planning and administration of the budget as well as the presentation or justification of the budget to appropriate groups or individuals.

7.4 The funding agency or administering agency shall consult with the head of its network library or machine lending agency before any action is taken affecting the finances of the program.

7.5 Network libraries shall work with administering and funding agencies to obtain outside funding for non-operational functions. Examples include grants and in-kind donations.

7.6 Network libraries and machine lending agencies shall provide all LC/NLS services at no charge to the patron.

7.7 Network libraries may provide supplemental services to LC/NLS patrons.

8. Planning and Evaluation

8.1 Network libraries shall develop comprehensive long-range plans, separate from state LSTA plans, designed to develop, implement, maintain, and improve services and programs and to optimize resource use.

    a. The long-range plans shall be developed in cooperation with appropriate constituencies, especially patrons, administering, and funding agencies.

    b. The long-range plan shall include measurable objectives and a timetable for accomplishments.

c. The long-range plan shall be developed in accordance with PL 89-522 (Pratt-Smoot Act as amended and extended – see Appendix D) as well as other appropriate statutes, codes, and legislation.

d. The long-range plan shall be produced in accessible formats and shall be advertised and made available to patrons.

8.2 Network libraries shall review long-range plans at least annually and shall assess progress toward meeting objectives.

8.3 Network libraries shall develop and implement methods for evaluating patron satisfaction at least every 3 (three) years. When patron satisfaction is evaluated, the results shall be used to improve services.

8.4 LC/NLS shall obtain consumer and network librarian input to its long-range planning activities and shall make the resulting plan available to consumers as well as to network libraries.

8.5 LC/NLS shall work with network libraries to develop and recommend methods for evaluating patron satisfaction.

8.6 LC/NLS shall develop and implement methods for evaluating network library satisfaction with LC/NLS services that include input from all network libraries at least every 3 (three) years.

9. Policies and Procedures

9.1 Network libraries and machine lending agencies shall have written policies and procedures for library operations designed to meet service goals.

a. Network libraries shall have written statements of policy for collection development and maintenance; for materials selection; for the reproduction of materials in accessible formats; and for interlibrary loan. Copies will be shared with NLS/NSS (Network Services Section).

b. Network libraries and machine lending agencies shall have written statements of policy for service provision to patrons including patron confidentiality and for patron behavior and library usage.

c. Network libraries and machine lending agencies shall produce upon request service policies and procedures in accessible formats.

d. Network libraries and machine lending agencies shall communicate any changes in policies, procedures, or services offered to other libraries, units, and NLS affected by the change in a timely manner.

9.2 Network libraries and machine lending agencies shall review their policies and procedures biennially.

9.3 Regional libraries and machine lending agencies shall consult with LC/NLS in the development and review of policies and procedures.

9.4 Subregional libraries shall include regional libraries in the development and review of service policies.

9.5 Regional libraries with subregional libraries shall include representatives of subregional libraries as advisors in the development and review of operational policies.

9.6 Network libraries and machine lending agencies shall provide staff and cooperating units with an up-to-date manual that includes policies and procedures.

9.7 Network libraries and machine lending agencies shall inform patrons of service policies and shall notify patrons of changes that will affect them. Up-to-date copies of service policies shall be maintained on fully accessible Web sites and provided in other accessible formats.

9.8 Network libraries and machine lending agencies shall develop or make available instructional materials in accessible formats to assist patrons in the use of this library service.

9.9 Regional libraries shall work with subregional libraries to develop strategies that contribute to a consistent range and quality of service in the geographic area served.

9.10 LC/NLS shall work with each region to develop strategies that contribute to a consistent range and quality of service for all LC/NLS patrons.

9.11 LC/NLS shall develop model policies and best practices and shall make them available online.

9.12 LC/NLS shall include patrons and representatives of network libraries as advisors in the development and review of policies that affect the network.

10. Reports

10.1 Network libraries shall maintain current and accurate statistical records to document use, services, and acquisitions; to meet the requirements of the administering agency, the funding agency, and LC/NLS; and to generate information for planning purposes.

10.2 Network libraries shall prepare an annual narrative and statistical report and shall make it available in accessible formats to the administering agency, the funding agency, patrons, LC/NLS, and other interested parties.

10.3 LC/NLS shall define, collect, verify, analyze, publish, and distribute comparable data for the network on a timely annual basis and shall make this information available to network libraries online.

11. Personnel

11.1 Network libraries shall operate under all appropriate federal, state, and local laws under a written equal employment opportunity or affirmative action plan.

11.2 Network libraries shall make every effort to advertise to, solicit applications from, and employ qualified persons with disabilities.

11.3 Network libraries shall maintain a commitment to cultural diversity.

11.4 Network libraries and machine lending agencies shall prepare an organizational chart describing clear lines of authority and reporting.

11.5 Network libraries and machine lending agencies shall develop and maintain a current position description for each title or each category of position.

11.6 Network libraries and their administrative agencies shall, at minimum of once every 5 (five) years, jointly review and determine staffing patterns and requirements based on, but not limited to, the following: long-range plans; demographics of the service population; geography; services provided; service patterns; physical facility; use of technologies; support provided by the administering agency; and the guidelines included in these standards.

11.7 The administrative head of a network library shall possess a master's degree in library science from an ALA-accredited program and shall be on the same administrative level as comparable unit heads within the administering agency.

11.8 Staff performing reader advisory service shall possess a bachelor's degree.

11.9 Network libraries and machine lending agencies shall plan and conduct formal orientation programs for employees that include information about blindness and disabilities that qualify individuals to use this service, as well as on the structure and philosophy of service.

11.10 Network libraries and machine lending agencies shall send appropriate staff members who have completed at least one year on the job to the LC/NLS orientation program.

11.11 The regional library shall provide training and orientation for appropriate subregional library employees within the first 6 (six) months of employment.

11.12 Network libraries and machine lending agencies shall encourage and support relevant continuing education activities for staff at all levels of the organization.

   a. Network libraries and machine lending agencies shall encourage and support staff participation in professional organizations.

   b. Network libraries and machine lending agencies shall encourage and support site visits and staff exchanges to other libraries as appropriate.

   c. Appropriate staff of network libraries and machine lending agencies shall participate in computer system user groups and other professional meetings and seminars.

11.13 Appropriate staff of network libraries and machine lending agencies shall participate in meetings of patron organizations.

11.14 Appropriate staff of network libraries and machine lending agencies shall participate in network conferences.

11.15 An LC/NLS network consultant shall visit new directors of regional libraries within the first 6 (six) months of employment.

11.16 LC/NLS will provide training materials relating to the operation of the new digital player to be used to orient new network employees and to update current employees.

12. Research and Development

12.1 LC/NLS shall conduct and encourage research and development efforts related to all aspects of this library service and shall serve as a clearinghouse for research and development findings.

12.2 LC/NLS shall collect and analyze data relating to elements of the standards for the purpose of planning and to identify quantitative norms for network library performance. LC/NLS shall disseminate the results of these analyses to network libraries and shall make these results available online.

12.3 Network libraries shall test, evaluate, and use new technologies, equipment, services, and materials to improve access to information and library services as well as to improve library services and operations.

12.4 Network libraries shall use compatibility and interoperability with local and national systems as criteria for evaluating and selecting technologies, equipment, services, and materials.

13. BARD (Braille and Audio Reading Download)

13.1 BARD shall be available to all eligible individuals, network libraries, and other eligible institutions.

13.2 LC/NLS shall maintain the infrastructure for BARD.

13.3 LC/NLS has the responsibility to add all new audio, braille, and braille music productions to BARD.

13.4 LC/NLS will ensure that a BARD site is branded for each regional/subregional library serving a state, as appropriate.

13.5 LC/NLS will provide and maintain training materials for network libraries to use in training staff in administering the service.

13.6 Regional libraries are responsible for administration of BARD, such as reviewing online applications and approving or rejecting patrons for the BARD service.

13.7 Regional libraries shall be responsible for first-line technical support regarding the use of BARD. LC/NLS shall provide higher level technical support to network libraries, upon request.

13.8 LC/NLS shall develop, implement, and maintain a process that enables network-library produced materials (audio and braille) to be loaded onto BARD.

a. LC/NLS shall develop and distribute guidelines for high quality network library production of materials.

b. Network libraries are strongly encouraged to follow these quality assurance guidelines.

c. Network-library produced materials on BARD that do not meet the LC/NLS quality assurance guidelines shall be clearly identified.

13.9 Regional libraries shall meet a one-business-day turnaround time to approve or reject BARD applications coming from currently verified patrons. If the applicant is not currently a registered patron, revert to the 5-business day turnaround time.

13.10 LC/NLS shall provide authorization for manufacturers of third-party players to enable their players to download and play LC/NLS books based on a formal agreement with the vendor.

13.11 Network libraries shall respond to approval requests for third-party players within one business day.

Guidelines

These guidelines, including categories, definitions, and target numbers, are to be used to determine appropriate and optimal levels. They assume a network library is performing all functions and meeting all standards presented. It is important to interpret and apply these guidelines in light of local conditions, such as organizational structure, the structure and philosophy of service, categories of staff and responsibilities assigned to specific titles and levels of staffing, and specific functions performed by the individual network library.

1. Personnel

1.1 Categories of Staffing

a. Professional librarian: Possesses a master's degree in library science from an ALA-accredited program.

b. Reader Advisor: Possesses at minimum a bachelor's degree from an accredited institution. The reader advisor works directly with the patron to determine reading patterns and preferences to ensure that individual needs are met. The reader advisor undertakes other duties as appropriate to enhance and support library services.

c. Paraprofessional: Positions that do not require a library degree, but may require appropriate degrees or certification in another field. Primary responsibilities do not include reader advisory service. Position responsibilities and qualifications are greater than those for technical support staff. Examples may include but are not limited to system manager, studio manager, production specialist or manager, information technology, technical services, volunteer coordinator, and outreach coordinator.

d. Technical Staff: Examples may include but are not

limited to equipment repair and maintenance, systems support, and production services.

e. Support Staff: Examples may include but are not limited to shipping and receiving, duplication services, and reception.

1.2 Levels of Staffing

A patron is an individual, a deposit collection, or an institution registered for service. FTE means full time equivalent. When a network library's number of patrons is not equal to the number in the guideline or its multiple, the staffing FTE will be calculated on a percentage basis.

1.2.1 Regional Libraries

 a. Administration
  1 full-time administrator

 b. Professional Librarian
  1 FTE librarian for each 4,000 patrons

 c. Reader Advisor
  1 FTE for each 2,000 patrons[1]

 d. Paraprofessional
  1 FTE for each 3,000 patrons

 e. Technical Staff
  1 FTE for each 2,000 patrons

 f. Support Staff
  1 FTE for each 1,500 patrons

1.2.2 Subregional Libraries

 a. Professional Librarian
  1 full-time up to 4,000 patrons

---

[1] Reader Advisor staffing may consist of full-time positions dedicated to this function and/or a combination of participating staff members who have reader advisory services as assigned duties.

b. Reader Advisor
1 FTE for each 2,000 patrons

c. Paraprofessional
1 FTE for each 3,000 patrons

d. Technical/Support Staff
1 FTE for each 1,000 patrons

2. Space

2.1 Guidelines for Determining Minimum Space Requirements:

Area	Minimum Size (square feet)	Comments
Reception	200	* Continuously staffed and properly furnished
Reading room	400	* Located near the reception area. *Stocked with catalogs, brochures, books, and magazines on cartridge, cassette, and braille. *Include tables with digital and cassette machines equipped with earphones for private listening. *Aids for eligible patrons.
Work area for clerical staff and volunteers	150-175 per person	* Space required for desks, patron files and records, automated equipment, passageways.
Offices	125 per person	* Private offices for at least the head and the assistant head. *Librarians and others may share.
Recording, duplicating, and storage	600	* Include space for recording booth, duplicating units, and shelving for master and blank media.
Shipping and receiving	1,500	* Includes a loading dock accessible to the postal truck.
Equipment and supply storage	800	* For storage of catalogs, brochures, and a 3-month supply of machines.
Equipment cleaning, diagnostics, and repair	500	* Should have adequate electrical outlets and network connectivity.
Conference room	500	* Should be available.
Staff lounge	300	* Should be available.
Book stacks	see 2.2	* Square footage required must be estimated after calculating linear feet of shelving.

Note: Network libraries located in the administering library may adapt the square footage requirement for shared spaces.

2.2 Linear Feet of Shelving Needed

Material	Maximum Number of Containers per Shelf (36 inches long, 12 inches deep, and 12 inches high)
Braille	12 volumes (for NLS-produced braille)
Recorded cassette (two deep, ends out)	98 cassette containers (7 across, 7 high, and 2 deep)
Recorded cassette (one deep, on edges)	24 cassette containers
Digital books (two deep, ends out)	196 containers (7 across, 14 high, and 2 deep)
Digital books (one deep, on edges)	48 containers

2.3 Reading Formats

	Circulated from:			
Format	LC/NLS	MSC	RL	SRL
Moon Type	x			
Braille (contracted)	x	x	only braille lending libraries	
Disc (33 1/3 rpm)	x			
TB and RD (16 2/3 and 8 1/3 rpm) and FD (flexible disc)	x	x		
RC (15/16 ips, 2- and 4-track)	x	x	x	x
DB	x	x	x	x
Music (recorded, braille, and large type) scores and instructional materials	x			

Glossary

The purpose of this glossary is to explain the usage of these words, phrases, and acronyms as used in this document, and by LC/NLS and the network libraries. It is not meant to establish standard definitions. The meanings of terms vary in practice and in various contexts.

Access. Freedom or ability to obtain or make use of.

Accessible. Able to be independently used by people who have disabilities. A fully accessible Web site, for example, is designed so that the site can be navigated and all functions can be used by a person who is blind or who uses an adaptive interface.

Accessories. Equipment used with talking book playback equipment to facilitate listening.

Agency. A public or private organization providing some form of service.

ALA. American Library Association.

Archival collection. Material preserved for historical record.

ASCLA. Association of Specialized and Cooperative Library Agencies, a division of the American Library Association.

Bibliographic control. A term which covers a range of bibliographic activities: complete bibliographic records of all bibliographic items as published, standardization of bibliographic description; provision of physical access through consortia, networks, or other cooperative endeavors; and provision of bibliographic access through the compilation and distribution of union lists and subject bibliographies and through bibliographic service centers.

BRA. Designation on older titles, with most titles only having one copy. Available in limited number of copies, some are thermoform, some press Braille. BRA 1 through 12999 are housed at

Multistate Center West. BRA 13000 and higher are housed at both multistate centers.

Braille. A system for tactile reading and writing devised by Louis Braille for blind persons in which print characters are represented by raised dots. The Braille system is based on a six-dot cell, arranged in two columns of three dots each, sixty-three possible combinations in all. The alphabet, numerals, punctuation marks, and a wide variety of symbols are represented by one or more Braille cells. Uncontracted Braille (sometimes called Grade 1) is written letter for letter, while English contracted Braille in the United States (sometimes called Grade 2) uses 189 contractions or symbols to represent letter combinations, prefixes, suffixes, or words which appear frequently in the language. There is also Braille for representing music, foreign languages, chemistry, computer, and scientific notation. English Braille, American Edition, adopted by the Braille Authority of North America, is the official code for Braille observed in the United States and Canada. Grade 3 Braille is an unofficial form of highly contracted Braille used by some students and professionals for note taking. Jumbo or large-cell Braille is a form of Braille using enlarged dots and increased spacing for individuals experiencing neuropathy or tactile insensitivity.

BRF. Designation for Special Braille Foreign Language Library Collection. Housed at the Multistate Center East.

BRJ. Designation for Braille titles formerly held by Jewish Guild for the Blind, primarily hand-copied. Most titles have one copy. Housed at Multistate Center West.

BRI. Designation for Braille titles formerly held by the Jewish Braille Institute, primarily hand-copied. Most titles have one copy. Housed at Multistate Center West.

BRM. Designation for braille music and books about music. Housed at NLS Music Section.

BRX. Designation for mostly hand-copied and one copy only titles. Housed at Multistate Center West.

Catalog. A file of bibliographic records arranged according to a definite plan which records, describes, and indexes the resources of a collection, a library, or a group of libraries. When provided electronically, often called an online catalog or OPAC (online public access catalog).

CB. Cassette book. See Talking book.

CBM. Designation for instructional cassettes about music. Housed at the NLS Music Section.

Circulation. The loan cycle of material from a library to the user and back. The number of items loaned during a given period of time is also termed the circulation.

Circulation transaction. The act of charging an item from the library collection to a patron for use outside or within the library and discharging the item upon its return.

Clearinghouse. A service for the collection, organization, storage, and dissemination of information and materials.

Consultant. An expert in a specialized field brought in by a library or other agency for professional or technical advice.

Container. A box or envelope manufactured to store and ship the cartridges, discs, tapes, braille, or other formats that make up a copy of the title.

Conventional Print. Material printed in less than fourteen-point type.

Cooperating unit. General term for the agencies in the service area that work with the network libraries in providing service. Those agencies may include administering and funding agencies, regional and subregional libraries, and machine lending and sub-lending agencies.

Cultural diversity. Representative of race, color, creed, sex, age, physical or mental disability, individual life-style, or national origin.

Demonstration collection. Library materials and sound reproduction equipment furnished by a network library to agencies whose clientele might include persons with disabilities. They are a vehicle for raising public awareness and advertising availability of services.

Deposit collection. A collection of library materials and sound reproduction equipment furnished by a network library to an agency with a number of eligible users such as a nursing home, a convalescent center, hospital, or library.

Digital book. A collection of electronic files, compliant with the ANSI/NISO Z39.86 standard, that presents digitally recorded material in a form that is accessible and navigable by blind and physically handicapped readers.

Downloadable. Material available for transfer from the Internet or a computer network to a desktop or other computer workstation or device. Examples include but are not limited to Web-Braille, Web-based audio recordings, and forms that may be printed and completed by patrons.

Electronic access. The ability to obtain or make use of information through a broad spectrum of electronic formats, devices, systems, or interfaces.

Eligible user. An individual who meets the established eligibility requirements for this service.

FD. Flexible disc. See Talking book.

Format. The layout and rules for transcribing materials in various media and the physical means used. In the latter sense, format may be used interchangeably with media.

Hardcopy. A paper printout of information, either in print or in braille.

HRLSD. Health and Rehabilitative Library Services Division of ALA. Superseded by ASCLA in 1978.

IMLS. The Institute of Museum and Library Services, an independent federal grant-making agency dedicated to creating and sustaining a nation of learners by helping libraries and museums serve their communities. Created by the Museum and Library Services Act of 1996, P.L. 104-208, IMLS administers the Library Services and Technology Act and the Museum Services Act.

Inspect. To check book containers for completeness and order of contents, damage, and foreign matter.

Interlibrary loan (ILL). The activity of a network library relating to requesting and obtaining, from other sources, materials requested by users.

Jumbo Braille. See Braille.

Large type. Material printed in fourteen-point or larger type.

LC/NLS. Library of Congress National Library Service for the Blind and Physically Handicapped.

Librarian. A person with a master's degree in library science from an ALA-accredited library school.

Limited-production material. Titles produced by LC/NLS in a small number of copies to provide supplementary titles to meet specific demand. Such titles are not duplicated generally for the network, but copies can be reproduced when the need arises.

LPM. Designation for large print music and books about music. Housed at the NLS Music Section.

Locally produced materials. Those items produced in special formats by regional or subregional libraries emphasizing user demand and titles of local significance.

LSCA. Library Services and Construction Act, enacted in 1962 to provide federal assistance to libraries in the U.S. Superseded by LSTA.

LSTA. The Library Services and Technology Act, administered by the Institute of Museum and Library Services (IMLS), and part of the Museum and Library Services Act of 1996. LSTA allows states flexibility in prioritizing their library needs and is the only source of federal funding that specifically targets libraries.

Machine. Specially designed playback equipment for recorded materials provided on disc, cassette, or other digital format.

Machine lending agency (MLA). An agency designated by LC/NLS to receive, issue, and control the inventory of machines and accessories essential to the provision of service.

Master. The original transcription of braille or recorded materials from which copies are produced.

Medium. Mode of transcription; braille, recording, and large type.

Moon Type. A system of embossed reading invented by Dr. William Moon in 1845. It was based on the standard alphabet and was comprised of fourteen raised characters used at various angles, each with a clear bold outline. Production of materials in Moon Type was discontinued in the U.S. in the mid-1960s.

National collection. Titles produced in quantity by LC/NLS for distribution to the network.

Network. LC/NLS and the agencies cooperating with it under the provisions of P.L.89-522 to provide library service to eligible users who are residents of the United States.

Network library. Regional and subregional libraries cooperating with the LC/NLS in the provision of specialized library services to borrowers who are blind or have physical disabilities. Also includes the NLS where it provides direct patron service (for example, with music services or to American citizens living abroad).

Outreach services. Library and information programs that seek out potential patrons, particularly those who do not or cannot make use of traditional library services or materials. Examples include bookmobile service, service to people who are homebound, books by mail, service to hospitals and institutions, and home visits.

Paraprofessional. Positions that do not require a library degree but may require appropriate degrees or certification in another field. Responsibilities do not include reader advisory service. Position responsibilities and qualifications are greater than those for technical or support staff. Examples may include but are not limited to system manager, studio manager, volunteer coordinator, production specialist or manager, and outreach coordinator.

Patron. An individual who or institution that is registered for and uses this service.

Print disability. Any disability that affects the ability of an individual to make use of standard printed text materials.

Processing. A term which may include everything that is done to a bibliographic item between its arrival in a library and its storage in the collection or may, in a more restricted sense, refer only to physical processing.

Quality control. Standards and procedures which ensure that braille and recorded materials meet LC/NLS specifications.

Radio reading service. Use of a radio station or the Internet to transmit content such as newspapers, magazine articles, current books, and other materials not available to persons unable to read conventional print. This service may be provided on a commercial or public service station, or more commonly on a side band licensed by a Subsidiary Communication Authorization (SCA).

RC. Recorded cassette. See Talking book.

RD. Recorded disc. See Talking book.

RDA. Resource Description and Access, "…a set of guidelines and instructions on formulating data to support resource discovery," developed "…to replace the Anglo-American Cataloguing Rules, 2nd Edition Revised." (http://www.rda-jsc.org/rda.html) MaRC21 is a machine readable format; RDA is a successor to AACR2. MaRC21 is the delivery method (a machine language), and AACR2/RDA are the rules.

Reader advisor. A staff member whose full time responsibility is to work directly with the patron to determine reading patterns and preferences in order to ensure that individual user needs are met. Possesses at minimum a bachelor's degree from an accredited institution.

Regional conferences. Geographic grouping of network libraries. The network is divided into four conferences: northern, southern, western, and midlands.

Regional library. A library for blind and physically handicapped individuals that is administered by a state library agency, public library, or agency for the blind. It must be designated by LC/NLS to administer services to the residents of a specific geographic area, typically a state. Usually provides direct services to patrons.

Selection. (1) A book title chosen to fill a patron request or substitute sent to keep a patron supplied with books if no specific requests are on hand at the time the books are sent. The latter service is given with the permission and wish of the user. (2) The process of deciding which specific tides should be added to a library collection.

Stack. (1) Frequently used in the plural (stacks), a series of bookcases or sections of shelving, arranged in rows or ranges, freestanding or multitiered, for the storage of the library's principal collection. (2) The space in a library designated and equipped for the storage of its collections.

Standards. Criteria by which library services and programs may be measured or assessed. Established by professional organizations, accrediting bodies, or governmental agencies, the criteria may variously reflect a minimum or ideal, a model procedure or process, a quantitative measure, or a qualitative assessment.

State Library Agency. An independent agency or a unit of another state government unit, such as the state department of education, created or authorized by a state to extend and develop library services in the state through the direct provision of certain services statewide and through the organization and coordination of library services to be provided by other libraries of one or more types. Also called library commission, state library commission, and state library extension agency.

Sublending agency (SLA). An agency designated by a machine lending agency to receive, issue, and control the inventory of specially designed record players, cassette machines, and accessories essential to the provision of service.

Submaster. First copy of a master; used to duplicate circulating copies.

Subregional library. A department or unit of a library agency that provides service to the blind and physically handicapped residents of a specified area of the regional library's total service area. Designation requires approval of LC/NLS, the regional library, and the state library agency.

Talking book. A recording of print material on disc, cassette tape or in a digital format produced for exclusive use of those individuals with disabilities eligible for the LC/NLS program.

Designations include (in alphabetical order):

33 1/3—A title recorded on disc at 33 1/3 revolutions per minute.

CB—A title recorded on a cassette at I 7/8 inches per second on two tracks of the tape.

DB—A title produced in a digital format and scheduled to be released by LC/ NLS in 2008.

FD—Flexible disc collection, 8 1/3 rpm, issued 1974–1994.

RC—A title recorded on a cassette at 15/16 inches per second on two or four tracks of the tape.

RCF—Special foreign library collection cassettes.

RCN—Network library cassette books accepted in the quality assurance program.

RCX—Volunteer-produced cassettes.

RD—Disc collection issued 1973–1987, 8 1/3 rpm.

RDF—Special foreign language library collection on disc.

TB—Disc collection issued 1962–1973, 16 2/3 rpm.

TB. See Talking book.

TM. Designation for tactile map collection available for circulation. Housed at LC/NLS.

Technical or support staff. Positions responsible for traditional library clerical functions as well as functions and activities associated with network services. Examples may include but are not limited to shipping and receiving, inspection and repair, production services, receptionist.

Title. The distinguishing name of a written, printed, or spoken work. By extension, the term is used to denote the work in general as differentiated from the variable number of copies of a book or magazine.

Trade book. A book that is produced by a commercial publisher for sale to the general public primarily through bookstores as distinguished from textbook editions, subscription books, or a book meant for a limited public because of its technical nature, specialized appeal or high price.

Union catalog. A catalog which includes all titles held by the network and by cooperating agencies, often provided online. Items produced through the network that meet LC/NLS reproduction quality standards may be deposited at multistate centers and will be so identified.

User. A registered individual or institution. See also Eligible user and Patron.

Weed. To select items from a library collection for discard or for transfer to a storage area.

Web-Braille. Web-Braille is an Internet, Web-based service that provides, in an electronic format, many Braille books, some music scores, and all Braille magazines produced by LC/NLS. The service also includes a growing collection of titles transcribed locally by network libraries. The Web-Braille site is password-protected, and all files are in an electronic form of contracted Braille, requiring the use of special equipment for access.

Withdrawal. The process of removing a title no longer in the library collection from the library's records of holdings.

Appendix A: Statement of Principles and Considerations

June 28, 2010

In 2005 the Association of Specialized and Cooperative Library Agencies (ASCLA), a division of the American Library Association (ALA), published the *Revised Standards and Guidelines of Service for the Library of Congress Network of Libraries for the Blind and Physically Handicapped (LC/NLS): 2005*. These guidelines are currently being reviewed and revised. A project director, a working team, and an advisory team have been appointed to develop a revised set of standards and guidelines to be adopted by ALA and published in 2011.

This statement of principles and considerations is the first product of this process. Rather than present the proposed revised standards and guidelines themselves, this statement is designed to enumerate the principles and considerations that will guide the work of the project director, the working team, and the advisory team over the next fifteen months as they review and revise these standards and guidelines.

Questions, comments, and suggestions are welcome from all stakeholders – patrons, librarians and library staff members, administrators, and all who have an interest in the provision of excellent library services to every eligible resident of the United States, as well as to eligible U.S. citizens living abroad.

Please send your questions, comments, and suggestions to the project director at the following address:

Tom Peters
TAP Information Services
6106 South Stillhouse Road
Oak Grove, MO 64075
tpeters@tapinformation.com

Principles and Considerations

Process

1. The standards are library standards developed by a professional library association (ASCLA, the Association of Specialized and Cooperative Library Agencies, a Division of the American Library Association) with the authority to develop standards for the cooperating LC/NLS network of libraries and their administering agencies.
2. The standards will be designed with maximum input from patrons and other constituents throughout this process.
3. The new standards will reflect the current and future environment rather than simply rework the 2005 Standards and Guidelines. The development of the new standards should not be constrained by the existing standards document.
4. Network libraries will strive to adhere to these standards and guidelines promulgated by ASCLA.
5. The standards will be applicable and usable regardless of library economic, legislative, and governance conditions.
6. LC/NLS will continue, through consultant visits, the follow-up reports, and other ongoing communications, to foster adherence to the standards by network libraries.

Scope/Content

7. The scope of the standards will cover all components of the LC/NLS national network: LC/NLS, regional and subregional libraries, multistate centers, and machine-lending agencies.
8. The standards will outline the responsibilities of the network library's administrative or funding agency, including but not limited to the financial responsibilities of that agency.
9. The standards will address changing service delivery methods employed by network libraries.

9.a. The standards will be mindful that the technological expertise of patrons covers a wide spectrum.

9.b. The standards will consider the changing methods by which patrons request services.

9.c. The standards recognize that many patrons may not be able to access Web-based or other electronic services. The standards will ensure that, as LC/NLS and the network libraries continue to advance service technology, these individuals are not left without access to materials and services.

9.d. The standards will take into account that services may be accessed by intermediaries, such as family members, caregivers, institutions, and others.

10. The standards will incorporate sufficient flexibility to accommodate emerging technologies.

Service

11. The goal of the standards will be to promote the best library services possible for all eligible individuals.

    11.a. The standards will describe quality library services that every eligible patron has a right to expect.

    11.b. The standards will be clearly written in language that is easily understood by all constituents.

    11.c. The standards will be available in alternative formats including braille, large print, audio, and electronic formats.

12. LC/NLS network libraries and their administrative agencies have the responsibility to use the standards for the improvement of service to patrons.

13. The standards will focus on the provision of services, while recognizing that programs and resources vary from library to library.

14. The purpose of these standards and guidelines is to enable LC/NLS and the network of cooperating libraries to be flexible in developing services and collections.

15. The standards will take into account that many network libraries benefit from the utilization of volunteers to supplement their resources.

16. The standards will consider opportunities for networking, resource sharing, and collaboration that result in process improvements while maintaining the same or a higher quality of service.

17. The standards will encourage network libraries to consider the resources, activities, and services available through public libraries as well as other local and state agencies, and how they can supplement network library service to eligible individuals.

Patrons

18. The standards will take into account the broad variety in demographics, needs, and interests of patrons.

    18.a. The standards will encourage network libraries to review patron demographics on a regular basis.

    18.b. The standards will take language diversity into account regarding collections and services.

19. The standards will address privacy considerations for patrons.

Administrative and Legal

20. The standards will reflect P.L. 89-522 (the Pratt-Smoot Act as amended and extended) as well as the Americans with Disabilities Act, Sections 504 and 508 of the Rehabilitation Act of 1973 as amended, the Chafee Amendment of the Copyright Law, and other pertinent local, state, and federal laws as applicable.

    20.a. The standards will continue to reflect the letter and spirit of P.L. 89-522 which states that blind and other physically handicapped persons who have been honorably discharged from the armed forces of the United States must receive preference in the lending of books, recordings, playback equipment, musical scores, instructional texts and other specialized materials.

21. The standards will include output measures where possible and applicable.

22. The standards will include quantitative measures where possible and applicable.

Appendix B: LC/NLS Service Eligibility Criteria

Eligibility of Blind and Other Physically Handicapped Persons for Loan of Library Materials

Eligibility for Service

The following persons are eligible for service:

A. Blind persons whose visual acuity, as determined by competent authority, is 20/200 or less in the better eye with correcting lenses, or whose widest diameter of visual field subtends an angular distance no greater than 20 degrees.

B. Other physically handicapped persons are eligible as follows:

1. Persons whose visual disability, with correction and regardless of optical measurement, is certified by competent authority as preventing the reading of standard printed material

2. Persons certified by competent authority as unable to read or unable to use standard printed material as a result of physical limitations.

3. Persons certified by competent authority as having a reading disability resulting from organic dysfunction and of sufficient severity to prevent their reading printed material in a normal manner.

Certifying Authority

In cases of blindness, visual impairment, or physical limitations, "competent authority" is defined to include doctors of medicine; doctors of osteopathy; ophthalmologists; optometrists; registered nurses; therapists; and professional staff of hospitals, institutions, and public or private welfare agencies (e.g., social workers, case workers, counselors, rehabilitation teachers, and superintendents). In the absence of any of these, certification may be made by professional librarians or by any person whose competence under specific circumstances is acceptable to the Library of Congress.

In the case of reading disability from organic dysfunction, competent authority is defined as doctors of medicine and doctors of osteopathy who may consult with colleagues in associated disciplines.

Residency or U.S. Citizenship

Eligible readers must be residents of the United States, including the several states, territories, insular possessions, and the District of Columbia; or, American citizens domiciled abroad.

Lending of Materials and Classes of Borrowers

Veterans. In the lending of books, recordings, playback equipment, musical scores, instructional texts, and other specialized materials, preference shall be given at all times to the needs of the blind and other physically handicapped persons who have been honorably discharged from the armed forces of the United States.

Institutions. The reading materials and playback equipment for the use of blind and physically handicapped persons may be loaned to individuals who qualify, to institutions such as nursing homes and hospitals, and to schools for the blind or physically handicapped for the use by such persons only. The reading materials and playback equipment may also be used in public or private schools where handicapped students are enrolled; however, the students in public or private schools must be certified as eligible on an individual basis and must be the direct and only recipients of the materials and equipment.

Appendix C: Lending Agency Service Agreement for Sound Reproducers and Other Reading Equipment

WHEREAS, under Section 135, a, a-1, and b, of Title 2, U.S.C., the National Library Service for the Blind and Physically Handicapped in the Library of Congress is responsible for planning and conducting a national program of bringing free reading materials to the nation's blind and physically handicapped residents; and

WHEREAS, execution of such program includes selection and procurement of reading materials and their distribution through a network of cooperating libraries and agencies; and

WHEREAS, pursuance of this program involves the loan to and use by blind and physically handicapped readers of reading material in a variety of nonprint formats and appropriate equipment for their use which is the property of the Library of Congress and is distributed by cooperating libraries and agencies; and

WHEREAS, _____,
(hereinafter "Lending Agency") is particularly suited to assist in the execution of the program entrusted to the Library of Congress, National Library Service for the Blind and Physically Handicapped (hereinafter "Library of Congress") in the state or region of

_____.

NOW THEREFORE, in order to cooperate in making sound reproducers and other reading equipment available to the blind and physically handicapped, the parties hereby agree as follows:

A. Eligibility

Eligibility, its determination and certification is specified in 36 CFR 701.10.

B. Eligibility Approval

The regional library, because of its responsibility for the ongoing provision of library service, is the agency responsible for final approval of eligibility within a state or region. Implementation, in area where agencies operate separately from regional libraries, will normally be limited to regional library review of applications which the lending agency has evaluated as ineligible. The lending agency, within one working day, will forward these applications to the regional librarian for review, signature, and return to the agency. Should the regional librarian judge the applicant eligible, the agency must act upon the application immediately upon its return from the regional library. Application for service may not be denied without the signed concurrence of the regional librarian. The Library of Congress is responsible for determining final eligibility at the national level and for resolving questionable instances of eligibility when agreement cannot be reached at the local level.

C. <u>Designation of Lending Agency</u>

1. The Library of Congress may designate, in coordination with a State Library Agency, Regional Library, and Machine-Lending Agency (if separate) for the Blind and Physically Handicapped, as many lending agencies in a state or region as it deems necessary to furnish expeditious service to blind and physically handicapped persons.

2. With prior approval of the Library of Congress and in coordination with the State Library Agency and the Regional Library, sublending agencies may be designated by the Lending Agency to assist in the distribution of sound reproducers and other reading equipment.

3. Any sublending agencies so designated will enter into a written agreement (approved by the Library of Congress) with the Lending Agency and the State Library Agency assuring all provisions of this agreement are adhered to. A copy of the signed agreement will be furnished to the Library of Congress for each sublending agency assisting in the program.

D. <u>Transfer of Sound Reproducers and Other Reading Equipment</u>

Sound reproducers and other reading equipment remains the property of the Library of Congress. Upon receipt of written instruction from the Library of Congress, the Lending Agency will ship all or any portion specified of unassigned inventory as requested by the Library of Congress.

E. Responsibility of the Library of Congress

1. Subject to availability of funds and statutory provisions, the Library of Congress will procure and distribute sound reproducers and other reading equipment and accessories to the Lending Agency.

2. The Library of Congress will instruct the Lending Agency as to repair and maintenance of furnished sound reproducers and other reading equipment and accessories.

3. The Library of Congress will reimburse the Lending Agency on a per purchase basis, for the cost of replacement parts actually required for equipment repair and not furnished by the Library of Congress , PROVIDED THAT the Lending Agency has first requested and obtained written approval from the Library of Congress prior to purchase.

   a. Request for said prior approval will indicate the following:

      (1) Item description

      (2) Item unit cost

      (3) Number of units needed

   b. Pats purchased by the Lending Agency will be invoiced to the Library of Congress on Form 73-43 with original invoices attached, within thirty (30) days of said purchase. Form 73-43, attached as Appendix two (2) to this agreement, is available in quantity from the Library of Congress.

c. The Library of Congress reserves the right to withhold said prior approval when it determines that indicated purchase parts or cots are unreasonable.

d. The Library of Congress will supply the following:

(1) Replacement parts for reading equipment used in the program;

(2) Replacement parts for equipment accessories used in the program;

(3) Replacement parts for repairing Library of Congress produced cassettes; and

(4) Specialized tools and maintenance equipment, provided their need can be adequately justified. In cases of doubt regarding the provision of any item mentioned above, the Lending Agency shall ask the Library of Congress for a decision.

4. The Lending Agency using the free mailing privilege will employ the United States Postal Service as carrier for the transportation of Library of Congress supplies, equipment, and accessories.

5. In cases where it can definitely be shown that a hardship exists at the Lending Agency whereby the program will suffer the Library of Congress upon prior written approval, will reimburse the Lending Agency for costs incurred for transportation of sound reproducers and other reading equipment. Costs incurred without the prior written approval of the Library of Congress will not be reimbursed. Requests for approval must be in writing and must include:

a. A justification as to why the Postal Service cannot be employed,

b. The cost involved per trip, and

c. The cost per article transported.

Invoices for reimbursement shall be forwarded to the Library of Congress within thirty (30) days of invoice date. In the event that conditions causing the hardship improve the Library of Congress shall be notified immediately.

    6.   The Library of Congress will provide mailing cartons for sound reproducers and other reading equipment.

    7.   The Library of Congress will not reimburse for state or local taxes included in cost of articles purchased.

F.   <u>Responsibility of the Lending Agency</u>

    1.   The Lending Agency will serve all persons eligible for service within the designated geographical service area.

    2.   The Lending Agency will have custodial responsibility for all sound reproducers, other reading equipment, and accessories assigned to it, and will take normal security precautions for their safekeeping.

    3.   The Lending Agency will maintain inventory control over all sound reproducers and other reading equipment assigned to it, and will provide the following information with reasonable promptness

        a. Number of machines received, date of receipt, and the number on hand awaiting assignment–by model number and serial number;

        b. The number of machines being repaired, model number and serial number;

        c. The number of machines assigned, providing access to location information by type of machine, serial number, and name of the person or institution holding the machine; and

        d. The number of accessories received, assigned, and on hand, by type of accessory.

4. The Lending Agency will make available all pertinent files to duly authorized representatives of the Library of Congress or of the General Accounting Office if requested.

5. Records relating to recipients of Library of Congress reading equipment are confidential except for those portions defined by local law as public information. It is the responsibility of the Lending Agency to inform the reader at the time he makes application for service of the extent to which the information provided may be released to other individuals, institutions, or agencies.

6. Theft of equipment will be simultaneously reported to the local police and the Library of Congress as soon as discovered.

7. Subject to availability the Lending Agency will assign and ship reading equipment and accessories to eligible persons within three (3) working days of receipt of an acceptable application and adequate information for service. When personal delivery of machines is furnished, delivery time may be extended to a period not to exceed ten (10) working days following receipt of application. Within three (3) days of the application's acceptance the applicant is notified of the agency's intention to deliver and offered the alternative of delivery by the U.S. mail.

8. Lending Agency may produce its own application form for use within its service area, however, a Lending Agency electing to do so will have such forms approved by the Library of Congress prior to use. No forms will require more personal or medical information than the official Library of Congress form, attached as appendix three (3) to this agreement, and all forms will include a listing of the entire range of sound reproducers and accessories furnished by the Library of Congress.

9. Lending Agency which is not a Regional Library will:

   a. Maintain effective liaison with the appropriate Regional Library in their joint effort to communicate with eligible persons and provide them with the best service possible.

   b. Notify the appropriate Regional Library of each new reader added and likewise of each reader being taken from the rolls, immediately upon completion of the transaction; and

c. Coordinate with and assist Regional Library in retrieving sound reproducers and other reading equipment and accessories from inactive readers.

10. The Lending Agency will repair and maintain sound reproducers and other reading equipment preferably through the use of volunteer agencies.

11. Completed reports will be submitted to the Library of Congress by the Lending Agency as required and in the time specified. Copies of regularly occurring reports are appendix four (4) of this agreement.

G. It will be the responsibility of the Lending Agency to instruct the readers regarding:

1. Reasonable care of sound reproducers and other reading equipment;
2. Free repair service and the procedure for availing themselves of it;
3. Transfer of eligibility, to another Lending Agency's service area when reader moves;
4. Necessity of notifying the Lending Agency when taking sound reproducers and other reading equipment to another Lending Agency's service area; and
5. Necessity of notifying the Lending Agency of changes of address, change of eligibility status, or desire to discontinue service permanently.

In the case of interstate moves, the Lending Agency from whose jurisdiction the reader has moved will notify the Lending Agency to whose area the reader has moved, and furnish copies of such notification of the Library of Congress and to the reader's new regional library. Notification will be accomplished on the Library of Congress form designed for this purpose. This form, appendix five (5) of this agreement, is available in quantity from the Library of Congress.

I. <u>Termination</u>

It is understood that this agreement may be terminated by either party upon six (6) months written notice. Failure by either party to adhere to the provisions of this agreement will be considered just cause for its termination.

J. This agreement is subject to annual review.

Accepted for:

The Library of Congress

_____
Director, National Library Service for the Blind and Physically Handicapped

_____
Date

State Library Agency (in states where State Library Agency is funding agency or program administrator)

_____
By

_____
Title

_____
Date

Accepted for:

_____
Agency

_____
By

_____
Title

_____
Date

Appendix D: Pratt-Smoot Act and Major Amendments

Act of March 3, 1931 (Pratt-Smoot)
An Act
To provide books for the adult blind.

Be it enacted by the Senate and House of Representatives of the United States of America in Congress assembled,

That there is hereby authorized to be appropriated annually to the Library of Congress, in addition to appropriations otherwise made to said Library, the sum of $100,000, which sum shall be expended under the direction of the Librarian of Congress to provide books for the use of the adult blind residents of the United States, including the several States, Territories, insular possessions, and the District of Columbia.

Sec. 2. The Librarian of Congress may arrange with such libraries as he may judge appropriate to serve as local or regional centers for the circulation of such books, under such conditions and regulations as he may prescribe. In the lending of such books preference shall at all times be given to the needs of blind persons who have been honorably discharged from the United States military or naval service.

Approved, March 3, 1931.
Chap. 400. Sec. 1, 46 Stat. 1487
71st Congress

Public Law 89-522
An Act

To amend the Acts of March 3, 1931, and October 9, 1962, relating to the furnishing of books and other materials to the blind so as to authorize the furnishing of such books and other materials to other handicapped persons.

Be it enacted by the Senate and House of Representatives of the United States of America in Congress assembled,

That the Act entitled "An Act to provide books for the adult blind", approved March 3, 1931, as amended (2 U.S.C. 135a, 135b), is amended to read as follows: "That there is authorized to be appropriated annually to the Library of

Congress, in addition to appropriations otherwise made to said Library, such sums for expenditure under the direction of the Librarian of Congress as may be necessary to provide books published either in raised characters, on sound-reproduction recordings or in any other form, and for purchase, maintenance, and replacement of reproducers for such sound-reproduction recordings, for the use of the blind and for other physically handicapped residents of the United States, including the several States, Territories, insular possessions, and the District of Columbia, all of which books, recordings, and reproducers will remain the property of the Library of Congress but will be loaned to blind and to other physically handicapped readers certified by competent authority as unable to read normal printed material as a result of physical limitations, under regulations prescribed by the Librarian of Congress for this service. In the purchase of books in either raised characters or in sound-reproduction recordings the Librarian of Congress, without reference to the provisions of section 3709 of the Revised Statutes of the United States (41 U.S.C. 5), shall give preference to nonprofit making institutions or agencies whose activities are primarily concerned with the blind and with other physically handicapped persons, in all cases where the prices or bids submitted by such institutions or agencies are, by said Librarian, under all the circumstances and needs involved, determined to be fair and reasonable.

"Sec. 2. (a) The Librarian of Congress may contract or otherwise arrange with such public or other nonprofit libraries, agencies, or organizations as he may deem appropriate to serve as local or regional centers for the circulation of (1) books, recordings, and reproducers referred to in the first section of this Act, and (2) musical scores, instructional texts, and other specialized materials referred to in the Act of October 9, 1962, as amended (2 U.S.C. 135a-1), under such conditions and regulations as he may prescribe. In the lending of such books, recordings, reproducers, musical scores, instructional texts, and other specialized materials, preference shall at all times be given to the needs of the blind and of the other physically handicapped persons who have been honorably discharged from the Armed Forces of the United States.

"(b) There are authorized to be appropriated such sums as may be necessary to carry out the purposes of this section."

Sec. 2. The Act entitled "An Act to establish in the Library of Congress a library of musical scores and other instructional materials to further educational, vocational, and cultural opportunities in the field of music for blind persons", approved October 9, 1962 (2 U.S.C. 135a-1), is amended to read as follows: "That (a) the Librarian of Congress shall establish and maintain a library of musical scores, instructional texts, and other specialized materials for the use of the blind and for other physically handicapped residents of the United States and its possessions in furthering their educational, vocational, and cultural opportunities in the field of music. Such scores, texts, and materials shall be made available on a loan basis under regulations developed by the Librarian or his designee in consultation with persons, organizations, and agencies engaged in work for the blind and for other physically handicapped persons.

"(b) There are authorized to be appropriated such amounts as may be necessary to carry out the provisions of this Act."

Approved July 30, 1966.

Sec. 1, 80 Stat. 330
89th Congress. S. 3093
July 30, 1966

Legislative History:

- House Report No. 1600 accompanying H.R. 13783 (Committee On House Administration).

- Senate Report No. 1343 (Committee On Rules & Administration).

- Congressional Record, Vol. 112 (1966):

    - June 29: Considered and passed Senate.

    - July 18: Considered and passed House, in lieu of H.R. 13783.

Appendix E: ALA Library Bill of Rights and Policy on Confidentiality of Library Records

Library Bill of Rights

http://www.ala.org/ala/issuesadvocacy/intfreedom/librarybill/index.cfm

The American Library Association affirms that all libraries are forums for information and ideas, and that the following basic policies should guide their services.

I. Books and other library resources should be provided for the interest, information, and enlightenment of all people of the community the library serves. Materials should not be excluded because of the origin, background, or views of those contributing to their creation.

II. Libraries should provide materials and information presenting all points of view on current and historical issues. Materials should not be proscribed or removed because of partisan or doctrinal disapproval.

III. Libraries should challenge censorship in the fulfillment of their responsibility to provide information and enlightenment.

IV. Libraries should cooperate with all persons and groups concerned with resisting abridgment of free expression and free access to ideas.

V. A person's right to use a library should not be denied or abridged because of origin, age, background, or views.

VI. Libraries that make exhibit spaces and meeting rooms available to the public they serve should make such facilities available on an equitable basis, regardless of the beliefs or affiliations of individuals or groups requesting their use.

Adopted June 19, 1939, by the ALA Council; amended October 14, 1944; June 18, 1948; February 2, 1961; June 27, 1967; January 23, 1980; inclusion of "age" reaffirmed January 23, 1996.

Policy on Confidentiality of Library Records

http://www.ala.org/Template.cfm?Section=otherpolicies&Template=/ContentManagement/ContentDisplay.cfm&ContentID=13084

The Council of the American Library Association strongly recommends that the responsible officers of each library, cooperative system, and consortium in the United States:

1. Formally adopt a policy that specifically recognizes its circulation records and other records identifying the names of library users to be confidential. (See also ALA Code of Ethics, Article III, "We protect each library user's right to privacy and confidentiality with respect to information sought or received, and resources consulted, borrowed, acquired or transmitted" and Privacy: An Interpretation of the Library Bill of Rights.)

2. Advise all librarians and library employees that such records shall not be made available to any agency of state, federal, or local government except pursuant to such process, order or subpoena as may be authorized under the authority of, and pursuant to, federal, state, or local law relating to civil, criminal, or administrative discovery procedures or legislative investigative power.

3. Resist the issuance of enforcement of any such process, order, or subpoena until such time as a proper showing of good cause has been made in a court of competent jurisdiction.[1]

[1]Note: Point 3, above, means that upon receipt of such process, order, or subpoena, the library's officers will consult with their legal counsel to determine if such process, order, or subpoena is in proper form and if there is a showing of good cause for its issuance; if the process, order, or subpoena is not in proper form or if good cause has not been shown, they will insist that such defects be cured.

Adopted January 20, 1971, by the ALA Council; amended July 4, 1975; July 2, 1986.

[ISBN 8389-6082-0]

Appendix F: ALA Policy on Services for People with Disabilities

http://www.ala.org/ala/mgrps/divs/ascla/asclaissues/libraryservices.cfm

On January 16, 2001, ALA Council, the governing body of the American Library Association, unanimously approved the following policy. The policy was written by the Americans with Disabilities Act Assembly, a representational group administered by the Association of Specialized and Cooperative Library Agencies (ASCLA), a division of the American Library Association.

Library Services for People with Disabilities Policy

The American Library Association recognizes that people with disabilities are a large and neglected minority in the community and are severely underrepresented in the library profession. Disabilities cause many personal challenges. In addition, many people with disabilities face economic inequity, illiteracy, cultural isolation, and discrimination in education, employment and the broad range of societal activities.

Libraries play a catalytic role in the lives of people with disabilities by facilitating their full participation in society. Libraries should use strategies based upon the principles of universal design to ensure that library policy, resources and services meet the needs of all people.

ALA, through its divisions, offices and units and through collaborations with outside associations and agencies is dedicated to eradicating inequities and improving attitudes toward and services and opportunities for people with disabilities.

For the purposes of this policy, "must" means "mandated by law and/or within ALA's control" and "should" means "it is strongly recommended that libraries make every effort to…"

1. The Scope of Disability Law

Providing equitable access for persons with disabilities to library facilities and services is required by Section 504 of the Rehabilitation Act of 1973, applicable state and local statutes and the Americans with Disabilities Act of 1990 (ADA). The ADA is the Civil Rights law affecting more Americans than any other. It was created to eliminate discrimination in many areas, including access to private and public services, employment, transportation and communication. Most libraries are covered by the ADA's Title I (Employment), Title II (Government Programs and Services) and Title III (Public Accommodations). Most libraries are also obligated under Section 504 and some have responsibilities under Section 508 and other laws as well.

2. Library Services

Libraries must not discriminate against individuals with disabilities and shall ensure that individuals with disabilities have equal access to library resources. To ensure such access, libraries may provide individuals with disabilities with services such as extended loan periods, waived late fines, extended reserve periods, library cards for proxies, books by mail, reference services by fax or email, home delivery service, remote access to the OPAC, remote electronic access to library resources, volunteer readers in the library, volunteer technology assistants in the library, American Sign Language (ASL) interpreter or real-time captioning at library programs, and radio reading services.

Libraries should include persons with disabilities as participants in the planning, implementing, and evaluating of library services, programs, and facilities.

3. Facilities

The ADA requires that both architectural barriers in existing facilities and communication barriers that are structural in nature be removed as long as such removal is "readily achievable." (i.e., easily accomplished and able to be carried out without much difficulty or expense.)

The ADA regulations specify the following examples of reasonable structural modifications: accessible parking, clear paths of travel to and throughout the facility, entrances with adequate, clear openings or automatic doors, handrails, ramps and elevators, accessible tables and public service desks, and accessible public conveniences such as restrooms, drinking fountains, public telephones and TTYs. Other reasonable modifications may include visible alarms in rest rooms and general usage areas and signs that have Braille and easily visible character size, font, contrast and finish.

One way to accommodate barriers to communication, as listed in the ADA regulations, is to make print materials available in alternative formats such as large type, audio recording, Braille, and electronic formats. Other reasonable modifications to communications may include providing an interpreter or real-time captioning services for public programs and reference services through TTY or other alternative methods. The ADA requires that modifications to communications must be provided as long as they are "reasonable," do not "fundamentally alter" the nature of the goods or services offered by the library, or result in an "undue burden" on the library.

4. Collections

Library materials must be accessible to all patrons including people with disabilities. Materials must be available to individuals with disabilities in a variety of formats and with accommodations, as long as the modified formats and accommodations are "reasonable," do not "fundamentally alter" the library's services, and do not place an "undue burden" on the library. Examples of accommodations include assistive technology, auxiliary devices and physical assistance.

Within the framework of the library's mission and collection policies, public, school, and academic library collections should include materials with accurate and up-to-date information on the spectrum of disabilities, disability issues, and services for people with disabilities, their families, and other concerned persons. Depending on the community being served, libraries may include related medical, health, and mental health information and information on legal rights, accommodations, and employment opportunities.

5. Assistive Technology

Well-planned technological solutions and access points, based on the concepts of universal design, are essential for effective use of information and other library services by all people. Libraries should work with people with disabilities, agencies, organizations and vendors to integrate assistive technology into their facilities and services to meet the needs of people with a broad range of disabilities, including learning, mobility, sensory and developmental disabilities. Library staff should be aware of how available technologies address disabilities and know how to assist all users with library technology.

6. Employment

ALA must work with employers in the public and private sectors to recruit people with disabilities into the library profession, first into library schools and then into employment at all levels within the profession.

Libraries must provide reasonable accommodations for qualified individuals with disabilities unless the library can show that the accommodations would impose an "undue hardship" on its operations. Libraries must also ensure that their policies and procedures are consistent with the ADA and other laws.

7. Library Education, Training and Professional Development

All graduate programs in library and information studies should require students to learn about accessibility issues, assistive technology, the needs of people with disabilities both as users and employees, and laws applicable to the rights of people with disabilities as they impact library services.

Libraries should provide training opportunities for all library employees and volunteers in order to sensitize them to issues affecting people with disabilities and to teach effective techniques for providing services for users with disabilities and for working with colleagues with disabilities.

8. ALA Conferences

ALA conferences held at facilities that are "public accommodations" (e.g. hotels and convention centers) must be accessible to participants with disabilities. The association and its staff, members, exhibitors, and hospitality industry agents must consider the needs of conference participants with disabilities in the selection, planning, and layout of all conference facilities, especially meeting rooms and exhibit areas. ALA Conference Services Office and division offices offering conferences must make every effort to provide accessible accommodations as requested by individuals with special needs or alternative accessible arrangements must be made.

Conference programs and meetings focusing on the needs of, services to, or of particular interest to people with disabilities should have priority for central meeting locations in the convention/conference center or official conference hotels.

9. ALA Publications and Communications

All ALA publications, including books, journals, and correspondence, must be available in alternative formats including electronic text. The ALA Web site must conform to the currently accepted guidelines for accessibility, such as those issued by the World Wide Web Consortium.

Index

Note: Glossary items are not indexed here.

Administration and organization: 29-30
ALA Policy on Confidentiality of Library Records: 14, 75
ALA Policy on Services for People with Disabilities: 76-79
American Printing House for the Blind: 1
American Sign Language: 77
Americans with Disabilities Act of 1990: 5, 58, 76
ASCLA (Association of Specialized and Cooperative Library Agencies): 3-5, 56
Assistive technology: 78

BARD (Braille and Audio Reading Download): 6, 15, 37-38
Battelle Columbus Laboratories: 4
Braille Book Review: 16
Braille, Louis: 26, 45
Book discussion groups: 19
Boston Public Library: 1
Budget and funding: 30-31

Caregivers: 57
Centenarians: 15
Certifying authority: 60
Chafee Amendment: 58
Children, services for: 2, 14, 19
Comprehensive Mailing List System (CMLS): 20
Confidentiality: 14, 33. See also ALA Policy on Confidentiality of Library Records.
Consultants: 26
Consulting services: 26-28

Deines-Jones, Courtney: 9

Demographic analysis: 26, 35, 58
Deposit and demonstration collections: 19, 30, 40

Formats: 43

Glossary: 44-54
Guidelines: 39-43

Hornung, Susan: 9

Interlibrary loan: 19
Internship programs: 28-29

Keller, Helen: 26

Languages other than English: 16
Lending Agency Service Agreement: 29, 62-70
Library Bill of Rights: 74
Loan periods: 15, 77
LC/NLS Service Eligibility Criteria: 60-61
LSCA (Library Services and Construction Act): 2
LSTA (Library Services and Technology Act): 31

Machine Lending Agencies (MLA): 15
MARC 21: 24, 51
Martin, Lowell A.: 3
MSCE Quality Assurance Program: 21. See also Quality assurance
Music services and materials: 19-20

National library collection: 23
Network-library produced materials: 37-38
Newsletters: 17-18

Orientation program: 35

81

Paraprofessional: 39, 40, 41

Patrons: 14-20, 58

Personnel: 34-36, 39-40. See also Staffing levels.

Peters, Tom: 55

Planning and evaluation: 31-32

Playback equipment: 15, 22-23, 32, 36. See also Third-party players.

Policies and procedures: 32-34

Pratt-Smoot Act: 1, 14, 58, 71-73

Privacy: See Confidentiality.

Project archive: 10

Provision of services: 14-20

Public education and outreach: 25-26

Quality assurance: 6, 24, 37. See also MSCE Quality Assurance Program.

Reader advisor: 16, 35, 39, 40, 41

Reading formats: See Formats.

Reading programs: 19

Reference requests: 17

Regional conferences: 30

Regional libraries: 1, 2, 4, 7, 21, 22, 26, 27, 29, 33, 34, 36, 37, 38, 40

Rehabilitation Act of 1973: 58, 76

Reports: 34

Research and Development: 36-37

Resource Development and Management: 21-25

Shaw, Ralph R.: 3

Shelving guidelines: 43

Space guidelines: 42

St. John, Francis R.: 2, 8

Staffing categories: 39-40. See also Personnel and Staffing levels.

Staffing levels: 40-41. See also Personnel and Staffing categories.

Statement of Principles and Considerations: 55-59

Sublending Agencies (SLA): 15
Subregional Libraries: 1, 2, 6, 11, 22, 27, 33, 34, 36, 40-41
Support staff: 40, 41

Talking Book Topics: 16
Technical staff: 39, 40, 41
Theft of equipment: 67
Third-party players: 38. See also Playback equipment.

United State Postal Service (USPS): 17

Veterans: 15, 61
Volunteers and Internship Programs: 11, 27-28

Web Accessibility Initiative of the World Wide Web Consortium: 18, 20
World Wide Web Consortium: 18, 20, 79

Young, John Russell: 1

www.ingramcontent.com/pod-product-compliance
Lightning Source LLC
Chambersburg PA
CBHW081211170426
43198CB00018B/2917